The Alternative

by

Martin Weisberg, M.D.

INFINITY
PUBLISHING

ISBN 978-0-7414-0212-7
ISBN 978-0-7414-9107-9 eBook

Published

INFINITY PUBLISHING
1094 New DeHaven Street, Suite 100
West Conshohocken, PA 19428-2713
Toll-free (877) BUY BOOK
Local Phone (610) 941-9999
Fax (610) 941-9959
Info@buybooksontheweb.com
www.buybooksontheweb.com

Dedicated to my father,
who taught me how to tell a story,
and my mother who claims she
taught me everything else.

Chapter 1

"Her pressure's dropping! It was fine a minute ago, in fact it was a little on the high side. Is everything going okay down there Al?" Dr. Arnie Geller was at the beginning of one of those infrequent rides that anesthesiologists both live for and hate. His patient was in trouble. Although a hundred percent of his concentration should have been directed toward the 37 year-old woman on the operating table, he couldn't help thinking about a conversation he had on the last day of his gynecology rotation seven years ago when he told his advisor, Dr. Alfred Dackel, that he'd decided to become an anesthesiologist. Not only could he hear the words again, he could also smell the combination of Royal Copenhagen Musk for Men, wet wool and fried whiting as they sat in the cafeteria that rainy Friday morning.

"A gas passer? Is that what you want to do?" exploded Dackel. "For Christ's sake Arnold, you're a good doctor, why do you want to waste your talent sitting on your ass and listening to monitors beep all day long? You know what they say about anesthesia, it's weeks and weeks of total boredom interrupted by occasional moments of sheer terror."

How right he was, and this was one of those moments. Monitors beeping, heart rates increasing, especially his, and all eyes on him. Trying to act calm, he said, "Hang on, children, don't panic yet. Let Uncle Arnie run in some fluid and give her a hit of this stuff. He reached up and turned the little blue wheel on the IV tubing flow controller and watched as the lazy drip---drip---drip of the sugar and saltwater solution quickened to an urgent *drip-drip-drip*, as if even the IV recognized the gravity of the situation. He injected a small syringe of medication that he always had within reach.

"Pressure's still dropping. I'm losing her. Get me some help! What the hell's going on down there, Al?"

"Nothing. I mean I don't think anything's wrong. The monitor's out but...I'm not really sure." The voice came from the other side of the drapes which were taped up to two IV poles, separating the anesthesiologist and the patient's head from the rest of the world.

The voice belonged to Arnie's old medical school advisor, Dr. Alfred Dackel, a relatively short, more than moderately stout and furiously balding, 58 year-old gynecologist who was not really sure what was going on. The truth was he didn't even have a clue. This was the first hysteroscopic endometrial ablation he had ever done. He had only just recently taken a two-day (really a day and a half) course where he learned the procedure which he hadn't even especially wanted to learn. He preferred the tried and true techniques of traditional gynecology. He knew how to perform one of the fastest hysterectomies at 14th Street Hospital and, by everyone's admission, one of the best. But times had changed. "Women are being convinced by the talk shows that hysterectomies are evil," he often said. "They want *alterrrnatives*." Whenever he said *alterrrnatives*, he said it with a nasal whine in his voice, mocking what he referred to as the "hairy arm-pitted, granola eating, in search of a meaningful experience group.

Kirti Patel, his young ex-associate, had known all the alternative operations, but she left him for a part time job at a local HMO clinic. She had two children and one cooking, and after just six years in practice she was burned out. She was tired of getting up in the middle of the night to sit with labor patients. She was tired of the long days in the operating room. But most of all she was tired of apologizing to everyone for the behavior of her asshole senior partner.

Al Dackel was cocky. He was also a male chauvinist, a closet racist and a vocal homophobe. But no one is completely bad. Al was an okay doctor who was actually very good at many things. He had lots of patients who loved him, and for good reasons. He returned their phone calls right away, he knew all their names and he always asked about their husbands and their kids. He was actually very kind to most of his patients, especially if they didn't challenge him. Of course he also had the ability to piss off any woman (and most men) by just being himself. Patel couldn't stand him any more, so she quit.

That left him alone, in solo practice. Solo practice was fine when he started out but times were different now. Solo practitioners were dinosaurs. Managed care didn't like solo practitioners. Some of the HMO's didn't even allow solo practitioners to participate in their systems. Luckily, Quality Health Maintenance, the HMO to which many of his patients belonged, did allow solos. Two days after Kirti left, they called to say that they wanted to come and meet with him to discuss his new contract.

They showed up two hours before they were supposed to. There were two of them. He was a 24 year-old provider representative named Brian O'Brien, a short, thin, delicate looking man with one of those haircuts that looks like somebody put a bowl on his head and shaved everything below the rim. She was a quality assurance nurse who introduced herself as Pinky Atlass, a woman approaching AARP age who looked like she weighed in at least 280-until she turned around. When she did you were obliged to add another 30 or 40 pounds to the estimate.

They started by asking to look at his patient records. "Absolutely not!" he objected. "These records are confidential. There's no way in hell I'm going to let you look at them, no way, never!"

"When your patients enrolled in our program, Doctor, they signed a release giving us permission to perform quality assurance checks on their medical records and to monitor their care," Brian said. "All insurance companies require access to medical records." Dackel heard a little too much *sss* sound in the word access making him instantly suspicious that he was dealing with a gay or at least a very effeminate male.

"Oh well, then be my guest," said Dackel spreading his arms widely and sarcastically gracefully, "but don't mess anything up." There was just a hint of swishiness in his tone and gesture, but not enough that you could really be sure that he was mocking O'Brien. "I'm going to finish up with my patients. Your appointment was for noon, I'll talk to you then."

Noon came and went. At 1:15 Dackel finished with his last patient of the morning. He closed the door to his office and took a fat-free bologna sandwich out of his briefcase.

"Damn that woman," he said to himself. "How can a person survive on plastic lunch meat?" He opened his Daily News to the sports page.

At 1:40 he invited the people from Quality Health Maintenance into his office.

"Let's get this over with," he said. "Where do I sign? You know I hate you guys. I think the HMO's are single-handedly ruining medicine. You're not managed care, you're managed cost! I saw how much money your CEO made last year. There's not a doctor in the world who makes a fraction of that kind of money, and you know who pays for this? The patients pay. They pay with their health!"

"Dr. Dackel," interrupted O'Brien, "we have a problem here. Your clinical records are not in compliance with our standards. As you know from the provider package you received when you started with us, and from our monthly newsletters, we require that your records include certain information, and that information needs to be recorded in a standard format. All we were able to find in your files are these 5x8 cards. Sometimes all you write is the date, 'normal' and a fee. You don't even sign them. This does not comply with our standards."

"Screw your standards and screw you!" Dackel screamed. "I've been practicing for more than 25 years and this is how I've always done it and this is I intend to always do it. I know what these records mean, and I'm the only one who needs to know."

"Dr. Dackel, I'm afraid that unless you agree to comply with our standards, we have no alternative but to not renew your contract with QHM, and....

"Listen sonny," Dackel interrupted, "I've been a participating member of QHM since the day you guys came and begged me to join, and ever since that day I have watched my income go down and my level of aggravation go up. I had a successful practice before you were out of diapers and I sure as hell don't need you now."

"Dr. Dackel," said Pinky, in a voice that was authoritarian yet soft, wise and caring, reflecting her thirty years as an emergency room nurse, "I've been in health care just about as long as you have and I think we're all frustrated with some of the changes that are going on, but times are different now. Please don't make any bridge burning decisions until you've had a chance to calm down and think it over."

Her voice was so soft and calming that he actually thought he could feel some of the fury leave his head and neck and pass through his chest and belly losing energy as it traveled like a storm going out to sea, or as he would have expressed it, like a fart in the wind. Her voice did another strange thing. It made his penis twitch.

What the hell is this? he said to himself. Am I actually turned on by this woman? He then mentally slapped himself on the back of the head and immediately put the thought out of his mind.

"What do you want from me? I'm an old dog," he said more calmly, "I can't learn all of your new tricks, especially all at once." He was frustrated, but he knew that they were right. He knew medical records were important. What if the patient moved or he retired? He knew that the next physician deserved all the information that was available. And what about law suits? He knew that good record keeping kept doctors out of court. He almost wished that he could start over again and correct all of his bad habits at once.

But then, as often happened, he couldn't resist his basic drive to be a jerk who constantly got into more trouble with his mouth than with his thoughts. "If you people can't be flexible, then throw me the hell out," he screamed as he swung his chair around and fumed as they let themselves out.

Two days later he received a registered letter informing him that his name had been removed from the list of QHM's approved health care providers.

Chapter 2

"Al, what's the matter Al?" Arlene Dackel asked her husband that night. She had a habit of beginning and ending most sentences with his name. She was used to him coming home from work, grunting at her, picking up the newspaper and flopping into his ugly La-Z-Boy recliner which didn't go with one thing in an otherwise professionally and tastefully decorated family room. But today, he didn't even grunt. He ignored the question.

Arlene was fifty-six years old. She overdid most things, her hair, her makeup, her clothes and especially her perfume.

Arlene never worked a day in her life and was proud of it, but that didn't mean she wasn't busy. She went to four different beauty shops (she called them salons). Every week she went to one for her hair where Mr. Lance exceeded the natural limits of teasing. Also weekly, she visited a different shop for her nails (fingers and toes). She had a waxing appointment at 10:30 A.M. on the first Thursday of the month at a third place, and every six weeks she took the Metroliner to go to a colorist in New York who managed to turn her hair a color not ordinarily seen in nature. There were those who thought it belonged somewhere near the red family. Others vehemently disagreed.

"Al, what's the matter Al?" she asked again.

"Nothing," he mumbled. They were a strange pair. If you'd ask either of them they would tell you that they loved each other and that they had a normal marriage, and if you looked at their relationship without considering intimacy, communication or passion, you would have to agree that they did.

They went everywhere together. They didn't fight because they didn't discuss anything important enough to disagree on. They had sex once a month or so, although it seemed almost like a chore for both of them. She didn't like to cuddle because it got her all sweaty and his body hair itched her. She didn't like to kiss either. She didn't like to kiss during the day because it messed up her lipstick. She used two different liners and two different lipsticks, one of which was the shade and texture of a yet-to-be discovered alloy. Then she finished it off with some sort of top coat. She didn't like to kiss at night because she used a special night treatment on her lips and the rest of her face.

Neither had ever been unfaithful, she because she thought it was wrong, and because she never had much of a libido anyway, and he because he was afraid of rejection, poor performance and getting caught, and also because he thought it was wrong. They coexisted well, and neither of them had ever expressed, out loud, the desire for more.

"Well something's wrong, Al" she said. "Al, something's not right. I can tell when something isn't right with you Al and I know that something is not right with you tonight. You're just not yourself and I know something's wrong. Al..." Arlene also had the habit of repeating a thought as many different times and in as many different ways as she could. When she ran out of different ways, she would start over again and she wouldn't stop until someone stopped her. "...Al, you can't tell me that everything's okay because I know there's something wrong..."

"Everything's fine," he muttered. " I just had a rough day. This managed care shit is going to destroy medicine. What's for dinner?"

"I made fat-free spinach lasagna with eggless pasta and fat-free cheese. I even found a marinara sauce made without oil, Al."

"Great—fake pasta, fake cheese and fake sauce," he blustered, "I can't wait 'til I have my fake heart attack."

"Al, that's funny, Al" she said, but not sarcastically. Arlene was one of the few people who thought Alfred was really funny.

During dinner she continued to talk and he continued not to. When he was finished he got up, still without saying a word, and he went to his chair. She cleaned up and went upstairs to read her newest Danielle Steele novel. She had a whole shelf full of them. One of Arlene's latest crises, which she spent the better part of an hour explaining to Dackel the night before, was deciding whether to store her books alphabetically by title, numerically by date of publication, or in the order that she read them. She hadn't yet made a decision so at this point they were thrown up there randomly.

When Arlene went upstairs, Alfred called his only real friend. His name was also Alfred, Alfred Klee, but just about everyone called him Red. Not Reds, because he didn't have red hair, just Red, short for Fred, short for Alfred. Klee was the name that they gave his father at Ellis Island. It was the best they could do to Americanize his original name which, properly pronounced, sounded like a bad cough. His father used to joke that they took the first two letters and the only vowel in the name and came up with Klee.

Red was also Dackel's accountant. They had grown up together in South Philadelphia. Each had been the first in his family to go to college. Each was now a successful professional. Both were jerks.

Red wasn't quite as arrogant as Dackel, but he was a lot more embarrassing to be around. If there was a wrong thing that could be said, Red managed to say it first. He wasn't a bad guy and he didn't mean to hurt anyone, but he was always saying the things that even most obnoxious people would just think but wouldn't dare say. He had no hobbies and only one real friend, Dackel. But according to his peers he was a damn good accountant. He also seemed to know how and where to invest his money and, as a result, he owned a lot of it.

It always amazed Dackel that Red had any clients at all because he always felt that he looked kind of sleazy. Maybe it was his hair. He slicked, gelled, moussed and fussed with it so much that despite the fact that it was all his, it looked like a bargain toupee that had long outlived its warranty. Or maybe it was how he unbuttoned his shirts with the oversized collars just enough to reveal a little too much chest hair. Or quite possibly it was just the way he looked at you that made you want to ask him how things were going at Allenwood, the federal correctional facility of choice for white collar criminals. To the best of anyone's knowledge Klee had never committed a crime, but there were those who were pretty sure that he had larceny in his heart.

"They fucked me Red," said Dackel, "They fucked me good." I just got kicked out of my biggest HMO. Can you figure out how big a chunk of my gross comes from QHM?"

"Sure I can figure it out, asshole," Red responded with a scatological sarcasm that men use when they attempt to communicate affection for one another. "You can figure it out too. All's you have to do (despite his college education, Red always said 'all's') is go to the report screen on that piece of shit billing program you bought and print report number 7. That gives you a breakdown by insurance company. But I can tell you now, you can't afford to be shut out of that one. I would estimate that you probably get a third of your gross from them."

"What will that do to my income?" asked Dackel, feeling his stomach twist.

"Well," answered Red after hesitating while he crunched some numbers in his head, "last year you grossed five hundred thou. Your expenses were about 240. That left you 260 before taxes. If you lose a third of your gross you wind up with about 330. Your expenses don't change, so your cut drops to about 90 thousand bucks—before taxes."

"Jesus Christ," screamed Dackel, "I can't live on that!"

"No shit Sherlock," said Red. "You better come over tomorrow. We'll see what we can do."

Dackel was beyond upset. He sat there on that ugly chair and cried for an hour. It was the first time he cried since his mother died. He didn't cry when his father died. He didn't know why.

Arlene didn't hear him. She took her shower and was asleep by 9:30. He didn't sleep very well. He spent most of the night trying to figure out whether he was a screw-up who got lucky and managed to get into medical school and make some money, or someone who truly deserved his successes who was just having a streak of bad luck. He finally fell asleep at about 5 A.M., but without an answer.

The next day was an operating day but Dackel only had two cases, so with luck he would be finished by noon. He called Red's office and arranged to meet him for lunch. Dackel often met Red for lunch, and it was a given that lunch meant Philly cheesesteaks, but there was always an animated debate about where they were going to get them. There are hundreds, maybe thousands of good cheesesteak places in Philadelphia, but two stood out. They also stood across the street from each other, Pat's King of Steaks and Geno's. Red liked Pat's, Al liked Geno's. They both grilled wafer-thin slices of some part of a cow in a lot of grease and, to add insult to artery, they topped the grease-laden meat with cheese—lots of cheese—real cheese (or cheese like material), not the fat-free grout that Arlene tried to feed him. The actual differences between the two places were subtle, but to a

South Philadelphia native that subtlety was what a good cheesesteak was all about. Each usually wound up each getting his lunch at his favorite place and meeting back at the car. When they were younger, they hopped up on the hood of a car and used it as a picnic table. But that was B.L. (before Lexus). Lately they just leaned up against the wall like the dozens of other future heart attack victims.

Today, Al didn't even say anything, he just walked over to Pat's with Red. "Boy, you must be depressed," said Red, you didn't even give me any shit about Geno's."

"Yeah," Al responded, I'm depressed all right. I'm depressed about the thought of living on ninety fucking thousand dollars a year. That's what I'm depressed about"

"That's ninety thou before taxes, crotch man," Red replied, using one of his favorite nicknames for his boyhood buddy, "but don't panic, I've been thinking about some options. Let's get some food."

They went up to the take out window (no choice - customers aren't allowed inside) and ordered cheese steaks "wit." "Wit" meant "with," which meant "with onions." While they were waiting, Red nudged Al and gestured with his eyes and a subtle, almost imperceptible movement of his head. Al knew what that meant and immediately but casually glanced to his left. He wasn't disappointed. A raven-haired twenty-year-old with a cut-up tee-shirt was leaning into the window. The crudely home altered scoop neck with the cut out sleeves revealed a generous helping of cleavage and small rim of left areola. "With luck," whispered Red, not as quietly as he should have, "and with just a slight change of posture, there is a chance that we may get to experience full nippleage."

A moment later, as if the god of perversion was shining his countenance upon these two social adolescents, there indeed was a shift and a momentary, but meaningful view of an entire unfettered breast, but not from the cleavage point of view. No, the boys lucked out and they got a clear shot, through the cut out armhole.

Red gave her a 9.3 because she had what he thought might possibly be a visible stretch mark. Al had really outgrown Red's rating game, but when he was with his buddy he usually played along for old times sake and because it was hard to explain to Red that he just wasn't into evaluating women with numbers anymore.

He gave her a 9.7 because he thought he saw a hair. The two friends had spent most of their adolescence and a good many of their pre-adolescent years preoccupied with breasts. Breasts were not so easy to come by in the post-war years. There was always National Geographic, but they showed native breasts and somehow it wasn't the same. There was also a "French Deck" of playing cards that Red found in the glove compartment of his father's Ford. Each card had a different pornographic picture on the back, but they were so old and faded that it was hard to see anything.

But then there was that special time of year when the boys knew they were guaranteed to visually score. It wasn't bare breast, but at the time it seemed almost as good. Late August, usually the second week, the newspapers ran the department store ads for back-to-school clothes, and they could always count on at least a half page devoted to "her first bra." Yes, pictures of four or five girls, around their age, wearing nothing from the waist up but bras.

They still both looked at underwear ads, but had long since graduated to Victoria's Secret catalogs. Dackel would leaf through them if Arlene happened to leave them around. Red called the company and had them mailed to his office.

"I can't figure you out," said Red, loud enough to cause several people to turn around, "you honk naked hooters all day long and you still go crazy when you catch a peek on the street."

"It's different," said Al, realizing that they were too loud and instantly lowering his voice. "I swear to God, they don't do anything to me in the office. It's just not the same, and I'm glad. Can you imagine how exhausted I'd be at the end of the day if I got turned every time I saw a breast!" In addition to that, if Al Dackel was anything, he was ethical when it came to sexual matters in his office. He never made a pass at a patient and he handled it very professionally whenever a patient came on to him. But, on the other hand, he sure liked it when he got to sneak a peek in a non-professional setting. "I'm still a guy, you know," he would tell Arlene whenever she caught him leering.

Actually, one thing did happen once that he was kind of ashamed of. He was examining a patient's breasts and he happened to glance up at the magazine rack, which had a Cosmo sticking out of it. Cosmo has a policy of having two consistent elements on every cover, direct eye contact and cleavage, and this issue had the best of both. There was Claudia Schiffer, exhibiting a giant economy sized cleavage and staring directly at him with what he saw as "I really want you" eyes. For a moment, and it was really just a moment, he imagined that he was David Copperfield and that he was practicing his version of slight of hand on Claudia's breasts. Dackel felt guilty about the incident for months.

Red and Al found a spot in the shade and proceeded to demonstrate the uniquely South Philadelphia art of eating a 14-inch greasy sloppy cheesesteak, standing up, and without getting too much on one's shirts. Eating at Pat's should be required training for all cocktail party guests, because if you can handle a Pat's, then miniature egg rolls and crudite are a piece of cake. (It's also good training for learning to handle cake).

"Boy these things must have a shit-load of fat," mumbled Dackel thinking about his coronaries while trying not to lose any of the very large bite he'd just taken.

"They do," replied Red. That's why you look like a fat load of shit." He grinned as Dackel managed to free the middle finger of his left hand long enough to salute Red. "Anyway, about this HMO thing, here are your options." He took a large bite, chewed it enough to get it to the side of his mouth and stuffed it in the pouch between his teeth and his cheek, kind of like a squirrel. "You can hang up the practice and go work for a pharmaceutical manufacturer or an insurance company. You can see if one of the hospitals wants to buy you out, or you can think about merging with another practice. Or, we can sue QHM and try to get you reinstated."

"Red, how long do you know me?" Dackel asked, but before Red could answer, he continued, "You know I could never work for anybody. I gotta be my own boss. How long will it take to sue them?"

"I dunno, a while," said Red, "but maybe we can get an injunction and keep you in until the case comes up. We'll have to check with a lawyer, but in the mean time you can start to rebuild your practice."

"I don't know, there's lots of competition out there and women are looking for female gynecologists. That's why I hired that Indian kid. She was good for business, but when she left, so did a lot of my patients."

"Well, I have a thought," said Red. One of my other clients hired a marketing consultant and her suggestions definitely helped. Let me try to find her number and I'll give her a call and fill her in. If she thinks she can help, I'll have her call you."

"I don't know," said Dackel, Arlene has a friend who used to teach kindergarten. She got bored, took three night classes in business management and now she calls herself a management consultant. She never worked a day in business, never managed a thing in her life, and now she charges two thousand bucks a day to tell CEO's how to run their companies. What the hell do consultants know?"

"Look, all's I'm telling you is that this babe helped my client out. If you don't want to talk to her, don't talk to her. Go back to the Catskills and get your waiter job back."

"Okay, give her a call. Hey, 10 o'clock," said Dackel. Red immediately knew that he wasn't referring to the time, but rather to a group of three teenage girls walking across the street in the 10 o'clock direction. "Look at the fantastic set on the blond. No bra!"

"Fantastic they are, but I disagree about the bra. You know some of the new ones let 'em bounce."

"Hey, who's the professional here?" said Dackel, cracking his first smile of the day.

"Yeah, whatever. I'll take her either way."

"Like you'd stand a shot at something like that."

As they rounded the corner and disappeared from sight and fantasy, Red brought himself back to his friend's problem. "I have one other thought," he said, "I'm not sure it will work. I have to check some things first, and I don't even think you'll want to go along with it, but do you know any shrinks?"

"Sure I know a few real good ones."

"How about a real bad one?"

Chapter 3

Dackel was upset and confused. Mostly he was scared. When he got into medical school he thought his problems would be over. He would never have to worry about making a living, he would be helping people, and his patients and the rest of the world would love and respect him. He didn't realize that he'd have to be a businessman, a personnel director, a contract negotiator, and a marketer. He also didn't realize that it would be so difficult to keep up in his field. Medical knowledge doubles every few years and it seemed to him that medical technology was exploding continuously.

When Dackel was upset, his body sent the anxiety right to his gastrointestinal tract. He was especially gassy this morning. He felt the rumbles in the car on the way to work and hoped they would settle down by the time his patient day started. They didn't. What was worse was that on this particular day his G.I. tract seemed to have an especially high sulfur content, which imparted that characteristic rotten egg pungency to his flatulence.

He had been in this circumstance before and it was a nuisance. He couldn't just go into the bathroom every few minutes because first of all, the bathroom in a gynecologist's office is almost never free and secondly because these were the kind of gusts that seemed to keep on giving—for a long time. Dackel had a technique that he engineered for occasions such as this. He would open his window, direct his desk fan towards it, and, when his intestinal pressure receptors told him he shouldn't wait too much longer, he would sit on his window sill with his butt hanging out the window and add his foul gas to the already not so pleasant Philadelphia pollution.

Unfortunately, in the midst of performing this moderately complex balancing act, he heard the words, "...in here?" and before he could get up, his door flung open and a woman he had never seen before walked in and started talking.

"Hi, I'm Deborah Metzger-Minkman." She was obviously embarrassed and somewhat bewildered. She also caught more than a hint of the fruits of Dackel's irritable bowel situation. "Alfred Klee told me to call, but I was in the neighborhood and I just thought I'd stop by and introduce myself, but I can see you're busy now, so maybe I'll just leave a card and you can get back to me when you have some time to talk." Within seven seconds, and without inhaling again, she made her statement, left a card, walked out and closed the door.

Dackel was mortified and besides, he hated hyphenated names. He hated everyone he knew with a hyphenated name with one exception. He thought they were pretentious and stupid. They made no sense to him. He didn't mind if a woman kept her maiden name as her middle name, but hyphenated names were another thing. "They are ridiculous," he would say every time he had the opportunity, "and those hyphenated babes who are the worst are the ones who made their children carry the hyphenated name. What if two hyphenated kids get married and want to carry on the tradition? Does that mean that little Miss Heather Beth Metzger-Minkman and her groom Zachary Brett Shapiro-Schnitzer would become Heather Beth and Zachary Brett Metzger-Minkman-Shapiro-Schnitzer? And what about their kids? Before long it would look like an Amway corporate chart with the great grandchildren never being able to enroll in school because the registrar's computer won't have enough RAM to enter their names!"

By this time he was usually on his feet, yelling and pointing his finger at nothing or no one in particular. He had nobody to yell at today so he just went through the tirade in his mind. He was sorry Arlene wasn't there. She liked it when he went off on one of his hyphen tantrums. She thought he was so funny. Whenever he started, you could see her trying to mouth the words along with him, "Heather Beth and Zachary Brett Metzger-Minkman-Shapiro-Schnitzer," And then she would try to repeat them as she laughed. Of course the names were different each time and she could never quite make it without getting tongue tied and laughing even more. On more than one occasion, she laughed so hard she wet her pants.

Later that day Dackel called the number. "Practice Doctors," the nasal voice answered.

"Debbie please."

"This is **DEBor**ah," she replied, putting a bit more emphasis on the **DEB** than the **or** but making it very clear that all three syllables were to be pronounced and making it even clearer that she was anything but a Debbie.

"Oh Christ," he thought to himself. "Not only a hyphenated last name, but a **DEBor**ah."

"This is Al Dackel. I'm sorry you caught me cleaning the window this morning. I know it doesn't look right for a doctor to clean his own windows, but believe it or not, I can't find anyone to do it. And how about the chemical smell in my building. Wasn't that odor something?" He was, of course, very unsmoothly trying to cover up the circumstances of their first meeting which ranked among one of the jerkiest moments in his memory, another being the time his tie somehow got between his speculum and his patient and, unbeknownst to him, he pushed it three quarters of the way into her vagina before she asked him exactly what he was doing.

"Yes Dr. Dackel," she said, knowing that he was lying. "As you know, "I'm Deborah Metzger-Minkman and I was asked by your accountant, Alfred Klee, to give you a call. I was wondering when we can get together so we can discuss what I have to offer and share some of my thoughts with you."

"Share your thoughts? How about sell your thoughts? How much is this going to cost me?" asked Dackel, with no hint of grace.

"Well that depends on your situation. I have several different fee structures. You can pay me hourly or we can work it so I get a percentage of any increased income you earn. We can talk more about it when we get together."

She sounded a lot like Fran Dresher, from the TV show, "The Nanny". Dackel thought Fran Drescher was the most beautiful woman on television. Ten years ago he ranked Meredith Baxter-Birney (the hyphenated name exception) number one, but lately, Fran was definitely the queen. They agreed to meet in his office the next day after office hours.

"By the way," he asked, for his own amusement, "Do you have a daughter named Heather?"

"No," she answered. He would have enjoyed seeing her tilt her head to the side and wrinkle her brow so that each of the wrinkles looked almost like the question mark she was trying to express. "My daughter's name is Emma Beth. Why do you ask?"

"Never mind, just curious," he said as he hung up the phone grinning. "Just as good."

He hadn't really gotten a good look at her the first time. She had only been there for a blink and she was wearing a raincoat. The impression that he had gotten of her however was that she wasn't bad. He reconsidered that evaluation when he saw her the next day. There was nothing horribly wrong with the way she looked, but a bunch of little things put her into a category Red liked to refer to as "no man's fantasy." She was in her very late forties, five four or five, maybe fifteen or twenty pounds overweight, with frizzy brown hair that had those phony henna highlights which, to Dackel, were less attractive and more obvious than any gray they were supposed to be hiding. She had a decent bust but a bad bra that made it look like she had four boobs with the two little accessory ones squooshing out of the top.

She also was in what he considered urgent need of a nose job both for cosmetic purposes to get rid of a major league speed bump and also to relocate her septum to somewhere near the midline. If nothing else it would eliminate that whistling sound she made when she breathed so she might be able to inhale without attracting dogs.

Still, she might have been considered kind of pretty except for her mouth. Even when her mouth was closed, her lips weren't big enough to cover her teeth. He assumed that either her parents must have considered orthodontia a frivolity, or perhaps her braces had been put on backwards.

She had on one of those sweaters with all the metal doo-dads and little mirrors all over it, and almost covering her ears was a set of industrial strength shoulder pads. He actually liked that look, but she wore a loose fitting floor length skirt and he hated that. "Too much clothes," he used to tell Arlene when she wore anything long or baggy. But the worst were the shoes, which he didn't see until she sat down and crossed her legs. Ugly heavy black lace-up boots that reminded him of the orthopedic shoes his grandmother wore. The only things missing were the holes on the sides that his grandfather used to cut out to make room for her bunions, which she called "my bunnies."

The thing that turned Dackel off the most though was the little bottle of spring water that she carried with her. It wasn't that hot outside and she wasn't in the desert. There were water fountains and sinks all over the place and a restaurant on every corner. Why the hell did she have to carry water around?

"Dr. Dackel, you have a lovely office," she said without really having looked around. "I spoke with Mr. Klee about your problem and he was kind enough to fax me some numbers which I..."

He cut her off. "Wait a minute Debbie." (He didn't call her Debbie on purpose, but he was glad that he did). "What right did he have faxing you anything? I haven't hired you. We don't have an agreement yet. That's private information. Nobody gets to see my books unless I let them see my books!"

"Well—I, I mean, I was under the assumption that you and he had, you know, discussed—agreed that..."

"We didn't discuss anything. He said you'd call me. That was it."

"Well, I'm terribly sorry and quite embarrassed, I just figured that..." and then she regained her composure. After all, she was the consultant, the expert. She had handled belligerent clients in the past. Even though he was absolutely right, she needed to take control again.

"Listen, Dr. Dackel," she said with a voice that she learned in an assertiveness training seminar, a voice that mysteriously seemed to be devoid of the nasal Nanny-like whine, "If you have any problems with what Klee sent me, why don't you talk to Klee. I didn't ask for any of this information, he volunteered it. Now do you want me to help you out of this shit pit you fell into or not?"

He liked that. He also hated her. Basically he was jealous. He wished that he could take command like that without exploding. He also felt a twitch in his penis. "Great, he thought, "Yesterday I see nipplage and jigglage with no reaction and today I get a twitch from a quadra-boobed whiny hyphenate with the nose of a prize fighting anteater."

"Okay, the damage is done already. So what do you suggest?"

"Well, I'm sure that Mr. Klee has gone over the numbers with you," she said professionally, although with the whine starting to return. "If you lose QHM, you'll survive, but you'll take home substantially less than you're taking home now. It will also effect your pension contribution."

Dackel always made the maximum contributions to his retirement plan. His goal was to pack away as much money as he could so that he could retire at the first possible moment. At this point, he had a little over a million in conservative stocks and fixed interest "instruments" as Klee liked to call them. He was aiming for two and a half million. That, he felt would allow him to retire without changing his lifestyle.

Unfortunately, Klee showed him some projections he had put together after attending a seminar in Phoenix, where he learned that because of inflation, cost of living increases and some other technical things that were too involved to explain to his client, he would need about 4 million to accomplish his goal.

"Dr. Dackel—Dr. Dackel," Ms. Metzger-Minkman said, a little louder than she had been talking, "Are you listening?"

"Yes I'm listening. I'm just waiting for you to tell me something that I don't already know. I went over all this for free yesterday with Red."

"Well, I was getting to that," she said, again feeling that she was losing the upper hand. "One thing you could do is to start a public relations campaign. I don't mean advertising. That's expensive and many consumers consider it sleazy for doctors to advertise. So we'll leave that to the cosmetic surgeons, but public relations is a different story."

"How so?"

"The talk show circuit, you know TV and Radio. Newspaper articles about you. Lectures at the library or in churches and women's clubs. You'd be amazed at the number of patients these things generate. It won't be instant, but I bet that with the right media placements, your numbers will be back to where they were within a year or so."

"How do I get all these 'placements' and more importantly, what do I say when I get there?"

"I get you the placements. I already do it for a lot of doctors and pharmaceutical and medical equipment companies, and we'll work on what you will say. Believe me, with the exception of one or two real doctors who do talk radio, most of these clowns will read right off the press release. Our main problem is to find you an angle. Do you specialize in anything?"

"Yes, good old fashioned, tried and true traditional medicine."

"Well, unfortunately, we're going to have to do better than that. Do you do any non-traditional things, you know, herbal therapy, acupuncture, things like that?"

"No!"

"How about natural child birth? No, that was more of a 70's thing. How about uterine conservation?"

"Uterine conservation? What the hell is that?" barked Dackel. Are you making that up?"

"No, actually, there is someone on the west coast who is making a fortune advertising that she can help you avoid a hysterectomy."

"Oh, *alterrrnatives*," whined Dackel. "I don't do *alterrrnatives*, and I suspect I'm probably too old to learn."

"Nonsense," Deborah replied, "You may be too stubborn to learn, but you're not too old to learn. All you need is one hook. One thing that will make someone want to get a second opinion from Alfred Dackel, M.D., the doctor on TV."

"I don't know," said Dackel, hesitating for a moment before sharing with her something that he never told anyone before, "most— most of these new procedures are done through scopes of some kind. You look at a television screen and do your surgery by remote control. I can't even get the hang of PacMan. I'm just no good at this new stuff."

"Al, take a course, try it out. Maybe you'll find something you'll be able to do."

"I'll think about it," Dackel said. "Now what's with your fee?"

"First you decide what you want to do, then we'll discuss my fee," said Deborah with a smile and possibly, yes very possibly, the hint of a wink. Another twitch, and she was gone.

Chapter 4

Dackel started out in pharmacy school but he never really wanted to be there. Ever since he was little, he wanted to be a veterinarian but his college guidance counselor discouraged him from even trying. “Veterinary school is the hardest graduate program to get into and frankly, I don’t think you have it,” she said, “and I wouldn’t waste my time applying to medical school either. You’ll never get in.” He took the Medical College Aptitude Test anyway, and scored in the “thank you for your application, but at this time there are no available openings” range.

He thought about dental school but he couldn’t carve chalk. In those days, when you applied to dental school they gave you a large hunk of chalk and a knife and you had to carve different shapes to demonstrate your manual dexterity and your grasp of spatial relationships. When he was a junior in college, Dackel had a friend who was a second year dental student. He worked with him for hours trying to teach him how to make chalk squares and spheres, but Dackel just couldn’t get it. In fact, he was so frustrated that he never even applied to take the test.

He considered podiatry school for a while, but he couldn’t stand the thought of working with feet all day. Sometimes he told that story at parties, on the occasional evening that he felt like being the center of attention. He especially liked the laugh when he told his audience that he ultimately went into gynecology. Arlene thought it was hysterical.

So he went to pharmacy school and did fairly well until he was caught trying to steal a microscope from the histology lab. The interesting part is that he was never really sure why he tried to steal it. Other than a few candy bars and a Papermate pen that he hooked as a kid, he had never stolen anything before. He had a decent microscope of his own, passed on by a cousin who used it in medical school and then shortly after graduation started a business supplying doctors to nursing homes and psychiatric institutions.

He was working in the lab by himself one day, he told the dean, and he just took it. He knew he couldn't sell it. It had the school's name etched all over it. It was just there and he took it. He didn't even hide it in a bag or anything. He simplify walked out with it, just as a security guard was making his rounds.

The offer was that the dean would not press charges if he left school. He hated it anyway so he took the deal.

He had no idea what possessed him to do so, but he walked out the door of the pharmacy school that day, got into his VW Beetle and drove 5 miles to a medical school, not the best one in the city, but nevertheless, a medical school. He asked for an application and filled it out on the spot, never bothering to mention his six months of pharmacy school experience.

Two weeks later they called him for an interview. One month later he got his acceptance letter. To this day, no one has the slightest clue why.

Chapter 5

"Dackel pushed the speed dialer button with Red's office number on it. His secretary answered and became instantly cold at the recognition of his voice. Not that he could blame her. He had done a stupid thing a few years ago. Darlene had been a patient of Dackel's and when she showed up with a case of genital warts one day, he called Red and told him about it, "...just in case you were thinking of shtupping her," he said, not realizing that he was on speakerphone. Darlene overheard the conversation and was furious. She quit on the spot. It took Red three weeks of pleading, apologizing and swearing that he would never breathe a word. It also took a $10,000 raise, but she did come back. Red also gave up his fantasy of one-day shtupping her.

"He's not here," Darlene said. "Would you care to try to leave a message?" He was tired of apologizing to her and he realized that she now lived to torture him every chance she got.

"No thanks." He hung up and called Red in his car.

"Well, what'd you think of the consultant?" echoed Red.

"Will you pick up the god damn hand set," Dackel yelled. "I can't stand that hands free."

"Is this better?"

"Yeah. She was okay, I guess. She wants me to learn a gimmick and go on TV and radio with it. I don't know."

"No, I mean what'd you think about her? Would you do her?

Red's view of women was that there were only two categories, those he'd "do" and those he wouldn't. He was also a master of rationalization techniques, which frequently allowed for conversion of those from the latter group into the former. A good example would be a statement such as, "Well she's fat and she smells, but I bet she'd really work hard to make up for it." Dackel was actually somewhat uncomfortable with the way Red thought about women, but he had to admit that even when he consciously tried not to, he too wound up categorizing almost every woman he saw into one of those same two groups. He often wondered when he'd grow out of it.

"C'mon man," Dackel said, "this is serious shit. She wants me to go on TV."

"It's not a bad idea Al," Red replied, "and I think I may be able to help. Meet me tonight."

They met that night at the Palm. They waited almost a hour for the table under Klee's picture. The Palm had caricatures of its best, or at least it's most well known customers. Klee was a big deal, so he got a picture, but it was not in the best spot. In fact, it was probably in the worst spot in the restaurant, right near the kitchen door. It didn't matter, Red wanted to sit under his picture and the ever-smiling maitre'd was always willing to oblige provided Red slipped him a ten.

"That's why they call it the 'Palm'," Red joked to Dackel. "Here's the deal Al," he said not quite whispering. "A few years ago I invested in a start-up medical equipment company, National Medical Innovations. What they did was basically steal the best techies from the successful outfits and put together their own line of stuff. They're just about ready to go with a new machine for treating women who bleed too much. They're just waiting for FDA approval. It'll be a matter of weeks. Meanwhile, they're starting to train gynecologists to work this rig, and if I play my cards right, I think I can get you in on it."

Dackel knew what he was talking about. All these new operations were becoming very popular. Laparoscopy, hysterocopy, harmonic scalpels, lasers, all kinds of new things that would undermine the reputation of, and eventually replace, the good old fashioned hysterectomy. A damn shame too. For 25 years he did 3 or 4 hysterectomies each week. He made a good living. His patients did fine and everyone respected him. At least that's what he liked to think.

"I'm not sure exactly what's involved, but at the board meeting they said that any doctor could learn it if they know how to do hytoskipy—hystoscomy—hyst...," Red fumbled.

"Hys-ter-AH-scopy, asshole, H-Y-S-T-E-R-O-S-C-O-P-Y," Al spelled. He loved to correct his friend who was always considered the smarter of the two. "Hyster is the Greek word for uterus, and "scop" means to look at through a telescope or something like that. When you put it together it's hysteroscopy. I can't believe you invest money in something you can't even pronounce."

"The stock just split 4 to 1," retorted Red. "Who's an asshole? But since you're so smart, tell me more about hysteroscopy."

"Hys-ter-AH-scopy, is an operation where you fill up the uterus with water or gas, I think they use carbon dioxide, and then you put in this telescope and you look around in there."

"How do you get the telescope in," asked Red.

"You are too stupid." He took the starched linen napkin from his lap and pulled out the Mont Blanc that one of his patients left in his office after filling out her registration papers. He started drawing on the napkin. A nearby waiter offered to bring him some paper, but Dackel waved him off.

"Okay, here's the uterus. It looks kind of like a pear, and a normal one's about the same size. Now in here, where you would find the core, that's the endometrial cavity," Dackel said, scribbling on the napkin. "That's the lining where the fertilized egg implants, and every month that lining prepares itself for a pregnancy."

"How do it know?" asked Red, quoting the punchline of an old joke about a thermos bottle.

"Estrogen, which comes from the ovary, causes this endometrial lining to grow and swell," answered Dackel after smiling briefly to acknowledge the reference to the joke, "and that happens every month whether or not the woman gets pregnant. If she doesn't get pregnant, the lining sloughs off and that's her period."

"I never knew that," said Red, surprised at the clear and patient manner in which his friend was teaching him. "But why would you want to look in there?"

"If a woman has abnormal bleeding, you know too heavy or too much or not at the right time of month, you can look in with the hysteroscope to see if there's any abnormal tissue, you know, polyps, fibroids, you heard of them, or even cancer. Frankly, I think you get the same results with a D&C, but a lot of the young hot shots say that this is better..."

"What exactly is a D&C? I always thought it meant dusting and cleaning." interrupted Red, enjoying his advanced birds and bees lecture.

"A D&C stands for dilation or dilatation and curettage. Dilation means stretching open the cervix with metal dilators, starting with very thin ones and using successively thicker ones until you get it stretched open to the size you need to put in whatever instrument you're going to use. Look here at the sketch. The cervix is the lower part of the uterus. Here, it would be at the stem end of the pear. Normally it's almost closed. You can barely pass a Q-Tip through it, but when a woman's ready to give birth, this sucker stretches open wide enough for the baby to pass through."

"Amazing!" said Red, taking the napkin and moving it into better light. But these people are talking about permanently stopping the period with this hysteroscope. I thought you said you just look through it."

"Yeah, they're talking about some kind of endometrial ablation," said Dackel nodding knowingly. That's where you burn out the endometrium altogether so she never bleeds again. The hormones are still there, and the estrogen still signals the endometrium to start to build up, but if there's no endometrium, there's no build up."

"Now its starting to make sense," said Red. "They were talking about a new way of doing what you said, but then they said that there was a lot more to follow. Look, let me try to get you into this class next month. I should be able to swing it. Christ, I put enough money into this thing."

"I don't know," said Dackel. "Like I said, I'm not much for this video game surgery."

"All's I'm asking is that you go down and check it out, Dack. It's just a weekend. Meantime, let's talk about the psychiatrist."

Chapter 6

About two months later at 6PM on a Friday, Dackel arrived at the Tampa Airport, on time and with a slight buzz. He wasn't usually a drinker but airplanes made him nervous and he always had a few cocktails when he flew. Although he knew better then to drive in his condition, he went over to the Avis counter, gave the stockholder his name and flashed his AMA and AARP cards for the discounts. The company had offered to pick him up at the airport but he liked the freedom of his own car. Besides, he had learned from the Internet that some of the best strip clubs in the east were in the Tampa area and he wanted to be sure he took in one or two during his stay. He had written down the names and addresses on one of his prescriptions.

Dackel was a "newbie" which meant he had only recently been introduced to the Internet. Normally he would have resisted getting involved with such new, hi-tech nonsense, but one of the pharmaceutical manufacturers offered to set him up for free if he agreed to attend a cyber-conference every month. The industry was always thinking of fresh new ways of bribing doctors to prescribe their drugs, and ever since the government stopped them from offering free golf outings to Bermuda, they had to do something. Dackel tuned into the first conference and slept through most of it. Then Red taught him how he could use his free modem and web browser to find dirty pictures and dirtier conversation and Alfred Dackel was fast becoming an Internet junkie. The name he used in the chat rooms and bulletin boards was "Goldfinger."

The weekend was courtesy of National Medical Innovations. According to Klee, they were an aggressive young company that was committed to living up to the Innovations part of their name. Red was right. They had been working on a variation of hysteroscopic endometrial ablation which was itself a relatively new alternative to hysterectomy. The word was that National had an entirely new approach, which if it worked, would introduce a whole new technology. Red called the chairman of the board and got Dackel invited to the first physician training session.

When he spoke to National's continuing education coordinator on the phone, Dackel was told that all he had to do was go down to Tampa and learn the procedure, get his hospital to fork over the nine hundred and thirty thousand for a complete set of instruments, and commit to buying all of the disposable supplies from them. Then, they told him, he could sit back and rake in the money. They would give him all the marketing material he needed, copy-ready mats for newspaper ads, brochures, referrals from their 800 N-O-H-Y-S-T-R hotline and placements on all the local television news and radio talk shows. They would even "media train" him so he would know exactly what to say during the interviews.

They would pay all expenses for the trip and the course and he would earn 16 continuing medical education credits. His hospital required 50 a year and he wasn't even close.

Dackel called Red. "My hospital will never buy a million-dollar-machine for me." Red told him to relax. He would handle everything. National was going to set up some test sites around the country and he would arrange to have Dackel as one of the investigators. He would also get a free machine for the length of the study. Once the hospital saw how much revenue it was generating, they would by happy to buy one.

He drove his rented Thunderbird to the Harmony Inn where National put up all thirty participants, and he checked into his suite. "Not bad," he said to himself, "a Jacuzzi, a patio, two TV's, a VCR, and a basket of fruit and, what else is in here, pretzels, candy, salsa and cheese. No tortilla chips." That's stupid, he thought, salsa but no tortilla chips. But, despite the snack faux pas, it was a very nice room.

There was a package on the desk, next to the fruit. He flopped down on the bed and opened it. There was a welcome letter from the president of National Medical Innovations, an invitation to a "meet the faculty" cocktail party that would be starting in forty five minutes, and a computer generated glitzy 1997 version of a "Hello My Name Is" name tag.

On the table was one of those "What to do in Tampa" newspapers. He immediately picked it up and turned to the last few pages where he knew he would find what he was looking for. He wouldn't have much time to himself, but it was rare that he got away alone and he was waiting for the opportunity to visit the strip joints that he had heard so much about. He went twice at home. Once he was immediately recognized by one of his patients who, at the time, was hanging naked from a pole at the side of the stage. Worse than that, the second time he found himself sitting two stools away was the father of a baby he had delivered two weeks before.

But out of town, he thought that it would be safe, or at least safer. There it was. The ad for Scampers, the place that his cyber buddies at Usenet alt.sex.stripclubs called the best in the country. Usenet is a collection of computer bulletin boards or discussion groups. Some of the greatest medical and scientific minds in the world share ideas and thoughts by posting messages or questions. Despite the range of subjects available to Dackel, the only two he ever looked at were alt.sex.fetishes and alt.sex.stripclubs.

Scampers was only about ten miles from the hotel according to the map in the information section of the yellow pages. He would go to the cocktail party, grab some dinner and then drive ten miles east to part with about fifty dollars in singles that he had been accumulating for such an event.

Again, Red couldn't understand why he seemed so obsessed with strip clubs when he spent ten hours a day looking at naked women. Frankly, he didn't understand it either. "It's just different," he would tell Red—and himself.

Alfred put on his white pants. After all, he was in Florida. He squeezed into a black Izod, stressing the tight knit to its tensile limits and hiking his pants up a bit so he could tuck it in. This shirt had fit when he bought it, but a combination of the fifteen pounds that he had recently put on and a rarely occurring event, it was a few sizes too small. The event was—and to this day, many people still don't believe that it happened— that Arlene actually did the wash herself. Of course she used hot water and put everything in the dryer for hours. He slipped one of his gaudy gold chains around his neck. Alfred knew that gold chains were not exactly the most current fashion, but he had no idea how really stupid this one made him look.

He brushed his teeth. Being well past the comb-over stage, he rearranged the few hairs he had left to distribute them as evenly as he could over what most people thought was an unusually large head. He hung the Do Not Disturb sign on the door before he went down to the party. It was always a difficult decision for him to make. He liked to hang the sign because he figured it would discourage a thief from breaking into his room, but it also meant that the turndown maid would not come in and leave candy or a mint on his pillow. Sometimes he called the desk to investigate the hotel's mint-leaving policy. But the fruit basket had some candy in it so, tonight, he just hung the sign and left.

The cocktail party was typical. Twenty or thirty doctors, most of them younger than he, several women and quite a few foreigners or "turbans" as he called them. Alfred didn't like foreign doctors very much, mostly because he didn't like foreign people very much. Although he didn't realize it, the other participants were all leading practitioners in the field of operative endoscopy, a technique that included hysteroscopy and laparoscopy. Many of them were department chairpersons and most of them were brilliant. He didn't realize how out of place he was and neither did the people from National. There were about fifteen National Medical Innovations staffers there. They called themselves technical advisors, but everyone knew that most of them were just salesmen. They all had perfect hair and big smiles. They all wore beautifully tailored clothes and scurried like new car salesmen to greet each new arrival at the door and offer a drink.

The buffet table was in the back of the room and Dackel maneuvered as if he was running a broken field play to get there without getting tackled by the "welcome to Tampa, damn glad to meet you" team. Touchdown! There was a bowl of iced shrimp. Number tens at least, he thought to himself, remembering his days as a waiter in one of the few non-Kosher hotels in the Catskills. That's where he learned that there were five different grades of orange juice and several different sizes of shrimp. Number tens meant that there were about ten to a pound. These were nice sized shrimp and, in his Catskill days, they would be served only to "A list" guests. How you got to be on the A list, he didn't know, but once you were there you got the number ten shrimp and the good orange juice.

There was also some fine looking quiche and a plate full of ramekins or romakins or what ever those chicken livers wrapped with bacon are called. In his home, he pretended to be on a low fat diet. His cholesterol was 256 with ridiculously high LDL's (the bad cholesterol) and barely perceptible HDL's (the good stuff). His wife cooked low fat for him and in the hospital cafeteria he usually ate only the "heart smart" food, but he cheated every chance he got, and when he was away he didn't even pretend.

In any case, he would be able to have his dinner right here and then head off to the club. He did want to get to bed relatively early though. He always found it hard to stay up during these all day courses. While loading up his plate he was approached by someone he recognized as Bill Davis or Jim Burns or someone with one of those generic names he never remembered.

"Hi Dr. Dackel, Pete Stewart, remember me?" Pete was the National rep who called on him at the 14th Street Hospital. He had stopped into Dackel's office earlier that week to drop off his tickets and an information packet.

"Sure Pete, good to see you," Dackel attempted to say. Unfortunately, during the "Pete," he launched a chunk of number ten shrimp fused with a cocktail sauce based bonding material to a fair sized piece of chicken liver. It bulls-eyed right onto Stewart's perfectly pressed whiter than white shirt, missing his silk tie only by threads. "No problem," smiled the man whose job it was to smile when doctors spit on him. "This will brush right off. I'll be back in a second." Stewart took off, probably to change his shirt and curse the fat bastard under his breath.

Before working for National, Stewart had been Dackel's Greco rep. Greco was a pharmaceutical company that had one major product, an antibiotic called Grecomycin. He remembered the first time Stewart came into his office with a portable TV/VCR combination unit. He played a six-minute tape about the new wonder drug and how it was the flagship of a new generation of antibiotics that cured almost anything without any side effects. He also told Dackel that he would be happy to leave the TV/VCR with him—indefinitely, just in case he wanted to show his office staff or patients "The Story of Grecomycin" provided, of course, that Dackel was pretty sure he would prescribe the drug when he felt it was appropriate—at least ten times a month.

This was just another creative way around the guidelines that the Food and Drug Administration and the rest of the government had instituted limiting the types and amount of bribery and graft that the pharmaceutical industry was permitted to use to entice doctors and pharmacists to prescribe their products. It was not as obvious as a golf weekend or a cellular telephone, although a few companies still got away with things like that.

Grecomycin lived a short life because a few months after it was released, it was discovered that it caused serious kidney disease in an unacceptable percentage of the women who took it. It had been tested only in men. Before withdrawing the drug from the market, the company petitioned the FDA to market it as "a man's antibiotic for man-sized infections." Fortunately they didn't buy it. They also rejected the statistical spin that women who took Grecomycin were less likely to require re-treatment with the drug. They based this on data that showed that very few Grecomycin prescriptions were refilled.

Dackel thought about all this as he wolfed down a few more shrimp—actually many more shrimp, and a few pieces of quiche. As he started to work his way toward the door, he heard the voice of a game show announcer. "Hi, Dr. Dack**EL**," said the smiling face behind the excessively affected sounds. Dackel immediately pulled off his name tag and put it into his pocket so no one else would stop him.

"It's **DACK**el," said Alfred, in a way that would turn a normal person into an enemy.

"Oh, I should have done my homework and learned how to pronounce your name before I introduced myself. That's one of the things you'll learn this weekend. I'm Dave Evans with Medical Media. I'll be giving you your introductory media-training course. I can tell just by looking at you that you're a natural for TV. Dackel knew he was lying, but he liked having his ass kissed.

"I'll look forward to working with you tomorrow and making the video on Sunday." Video? Alfred thought, What kind of video? But he didn't say anything because he figured it was explained in the information package that Pete whatever his name is had dropped off in his office. He hadn't read it yet. He had glanced at the contents, and recalled that they included a course syllabus, a three page description of the procedure he was going to learn, a five page monograph entitled "Introduction to Hysteroscopy," and a twenty two page booklet entitled "Marketing Your Practice."

He brought them to read on the plane, but he saw Howard Stern's book in paperback at the airport bookstore and he figured he'd read that instead. His wife hated Howard Stern and, when he was with her, he pretended that he did too. He wasn't sure why.

"Sure," Dackel said, see you tomorrow. He took the slip of paper with the list of the strip clubs from his pocket and glanced at the address of Scampers, which he had circled. Then he slipped out the door, skillfully avoiding Skip somebody and Bud somebody else.

Unfolding the map he had ripped out of the phone book, he held it under the map light in the T-Bird and memorized the few turns he would have to make to get to Scampers, the club rated highest by a an Internet guru who called himself Couchman. He pulled out of the hotel parking lot and went the wrong way for about six miles before he figured it out.

By the time he got to Scampers his heart was racing. He thought again about why he was so excited to pay to see what women paid him to look at—and touch and, as usual, the only thing he could come up with was that it was just different. He paid his six dollar cover and entered into the world of naked women, loud music and cigarette smoke.

He had only been in a strip club or gentleman's club, as they called them, a few times before. They had been pretty classy places, lavishly decorated and patronized by men in business suits. This one was smaller and not as well appointed. There were about 15 guys, none in suits, sitting around the two stages. Most of them were younger than he, and all of them were hipper. The music was metal and loud, and the room was smoky.

He took a seat between two biker-looking guys, ordered a white wine spritzer and took out a wad of singles. The dancer on the stage was a tall thin Hispanic girl with a cocoa complexion. Her breast implants were obviously put in by a doctor who needed a little more experience, but she was graceful and beautiful. She did all the usual things they teach in gentleman's club dancing 101: Self breast licking; private part rubbing; undulating; and open mouth puckering while pretending to say "oooh."

Most of the patrons seemed bored. Dackel loved it. He applauded when she finished her first song. No one else did. She came over to him and held out the elastic on her g-string while he slipped in a dollar bill folded lengthwise. She turned around, bent over and pulled the g-string away. Dackel shoved another dollar between her cheeks. She pointed to her cleavage and held her breasts apart while he folded another dollar bill. As he was depositing the bill, she pushed her breasts together trapping his hand for a few seconds. She blew him a kiss and slithered away.

Dackel pondered the unanswerable question again. Just hours ago thirty women paid him ninety dollars each for him to touch their breasts and their vaginas and anything else he wanted to, and it was work. Today it costs him a dollar for the opportunity to cop a two-second feel. He couldn't figure it out. He could never figure it out.

The next dancer was introduced as Angel. She was kind of plain for a stripper. She started her dance fully dressed in what looked like a parochial school outfit complete with saddle shoes and bobby sox. She wore her blond hair in two cute little pigtails, and she wore glasses. The DJ was playing "Girls Just Want to Have Fun." Dackel was having fun.

When the second song started, she took off her skirt and blouse. Instead of typical sequins and lace, she wore a plain bra and cotton bikini panties. For the first time that night Alfred got an erection, not just a twitch, but a solid woody. He got to see lots of naked women in his office, but her never got to see them undress or walk around in their underwear.

She started to make the rounds of the men at the bar. Some of them slipped her a buck, some didn't even seem to acknowledge her. Dackel held his dollar high above his head, straining his arm like Horshack when he wanted Mr. Cotter's attention. She came over and stared into his eyes for a full 15 seconds. She then looked directly at his crotch for what seem to him like an hour, but was really about five seconds.

"Would you like to unhook my bra?" she whispered in his ear.

"Sure," he said, loud enough to turn some heads. He was so uncool.

"Go ahead it's hooked in the front."

He fumbled a bit until he was able to figure out the mechanics of the device, but he was ultimately successful in unfettering two of the most beautiful breasts he had ever remembered seeing. And, to his trained and professional eye, these were 100% natural God-given breasts and breast byproducts with no artificial ingredients, preservatives or additives.

"They're perfect," he said. "Absolutely perfect." He based his evaluation on size, shape, contour (or is that the same as shape?), nipple configuration, areolar color, lack of blemishes, and overall aesthetic value.

Even Red would have given them a 10, he thought.
He gave her 7 or 8 dollar bills and she wiggled her way over to the next customer.

The next time she danced by him, she had taken off her panties and was wearing only the wispiest of g-strings. He had a wad of dollars in each hand and was waving them furiously. She pulled out the top of her thong further than the first dancer had. In fact, he was able to get a pretty good look at her perfectly hairless vulva. He stuffed all the money he was holding in his right hand into her thong.

"Slow up handsome, take your time in there," she said with a wink.

A high voltage shock went from his ears right down to his penis. He almost had an accident right then and there, but he didn't. She kissed him on the top of his head and whispered, "see you later."

When she was through on the stage, she came right over to Dackel, not even stopping to talk to any of the other men.

"What's your name, good looking?" she purred.

"I'm Dr. Alfred Dackel. I'm a gynecologist from Philadelphia." Dackel may have been the only human to ever gave his real name and occupation in a strip club.

"Well Dr. Alfred Dackel, I think you're cute, and I just wanted to thank you for letting me know how much you appreciated my dancing. Would you like me to do a private dance for you?"

"Sure, I mean I'm not sure. How much are dances?"

"Ten dollars at the table and twenty in the VIP couch room."

"Sure," he said, not really knowing what he was about to experience. He did have all kinds of fantasies and some good Internet information and, from what he understood, this was one of the most liberal clubs around. If his information was correct, touching was allowed. The girls were permitted to do whatever they wanted as long as you kept your pants on. The other clubs he had been to had strict "no touching" policies.

"Good, let's go to the couch room," she said with a wink.

She took his hand and led him up three stairs into a dark room. On the way she asked him if he was married. He answered honestly and didn't ask her any questions.

The VIP room looked more like an R.I.P. room to Dackel. It reminded him of a funeral parlor with thick dark maroon rugs, overstuffed sofas and that eerie smell of roses that overtakes you when you walk into a viewing.

She guided him by the hand to a couch in the corner and sat down next to him.

"I'm really not supposed to be in here," she giggled. I'm just auditioning here tonight and tomorrow and we're not supposed to do private dances, but the manager is a friend of mine and he said it would be okay just this once. Would you like some champagne?"

"Not really," said Dackel, "I'm not much of a drinker. But feel free to have some yourself."

"Alfred, you are new to this, aren't you. You're so sweet, I just can't take advantage of you. Don't you know that the champagne is overpriced and sometimes watered down in these places? It's a rip off. Forget the drinks. I want to dance for you."

She stood up, took his hands and put them by his sides. She lifted each of his legs and positioned them far apart.

"Now you just stay in this position honey, and I'll do the rest. There are some new rules here since the city council has been cracking down, but I don't think you'll be disappointed."

She quickly and unceremoniously took off everything except her g-string and started to move as sensually as he'd ever imagined a person could move. He sat there, legs apart, hands to his sides while she moved between his legs, teasing but never touching. She came as close to touching him as humanly possible, but without actually making contact. She brushed her hair against his face and blew in his ear. At the end of the song, she gave him a hug and pressed her pelvis against his.

"Want to go again?" she teased, "I was just getting warmed up." She winked at him.

"This is definitely not cheating," he meant to say to himself, but accidentally said out loud. "I'm not doing a thing. I'm just sitting here. It's not an affair, we're not having sex. This is just for fun. It's like the massages Arlene gets from that blind masseur. That's not cheating and neither is this. Sure let's go again."

"You're so cute," she said smiling.

The second dance was much like the first except every once in a while she would brush her knee against his crotch. At one point she was dancing with her back to him and pretending to grind her butt on his lap. She got a little too close, and made contact, and she stayed there just a little too long for it to have been accidental. Then she lowered her head to his lap and opened her mouth as if she was about to put it around his penis, but she never did. If she had, it would have been a first for Dackel. Although he had never admitted it, not even to Red, Dackel had never had a blowjob. He hadn't had very much sexual experience before he married Arlene. She'd never offered and he'd always been too embarrassed to ask. Often he'd wished that she would spontaneously just do it, but she never did. Anyway, this was the closest he'd ever gotten to oral sex and he was very aroused. At one point, he started to stroke her thigh a little too high.

"No, no, bad boy. You're not allowed to touch. Big brother is watching." She pointed to the corner of the room. Dackel looked over but didn't see anything. He didn't know that there were cameras all around the club for security purposes. If any of the patrons got too frisky, the bouncers would get a message in their earpieces and they would be on the guy in seconds.

The song was over. She got dressed in her school girl outfit, hugged him a little tighter than the last time and said she'd see him later. He paid her the forty dollars and gave her an extra ten. As she was leaving Dackel said, "wait a minute, how about another?"

"You're so sweet," she answered, "but I have a feeling you've had enough tonight."

She was right. He'd had enough. He was starting to think about things he shouldn't have been thinking about. Besides it was almost 11:30 and he had to get up early in the morning for the course. Still, he hung around for another half-hour. The girls continued to come around, he would give them a buck or two, but he kept looking for Angel. She never returned. He finally went up to one of the bouncers, a guy who looked like Popeye's archenemy Bluto (or Brutus in the later cartoons.)

"Do you know if Angel is coming back on tonight?"

"Tonight's audition night, buddy. She was just trying out."

"Do you know where I can find her?"

"'Fraid not, Buddy."

Dackel felt an instant emptiness. He didn't know why. He wasn't looking for an affair. He also didn't want to risk getting a sexually transmitted disease from a one-nighter. He didn't even have time to take her to dinner. All he knew is that she called him handsome, she looked at him in a special way, and she looked like she enjoyed it when he put his hand down her pants.

He paid his bar tab, nineteen bucks for two diet Cokes and a barely alcoholic wine spritzer, and left the club. As he walked towards his car in the humid, steamy, after-the-rain Florida air, a white Jeep Grand Cherokee drove up. When the driver rolled down the window, his heart skipped. For a moment he thought it was going to stop altogether. It was Angel's voice. He couldn't see her until she turned on the interior lights. Her hair was short and brown. She was wearing jeans and a T-shirt with what he assumed was the name of a rock group he never heard of. She looked like a typical college student, and not an especially sexy one.

"Hi," she said smiling.

"Hi," he blushed. I-I didn't recognize you— the hair and..."

"Oh, the blond wig," she said holding up a wig box, "I almost forgot. Need a lift?"

"No thanks, I have a rental."

"How about a cup of coffee," she asked. "There's a Denny's right across the road."

He looked at his watch but his brain didn't even register the time. "Sure," he said, "but it will have to be a quickie."

They both drove across the highway and parked side by side in the Denny's parking lot. As they were walking into the restaurant, she took his arm and led him to a booth next to the window. They both ordered decaf.

Dr. Dackel, I hope you don't consider this too forward of me, but there is something about you that made me instantly trust you. My real name is Carrie Bradford and I'm a drama student. I'm trying to get a job dancing to earn money for school. I really don't want to be doing this, but it's the only way I can think of to earn enough for tuition in the fall. I also have a problem. I might be pregnant. I broke up with my boyfriend last month. I'm ten days late and I don't know what to do.

"Have you done a test?" he asked.

"A pregnancy test? No, I've been afraid and I'm not sure I'll do it right."

"Oh, it's easy. We can do it right now if you want. Is there a 24 hour pharmacy open around here?"

"I don't think so, but Dr. Dackel, what if it's positive?"

"Why don't we jump off that bridge when we come to it," he said, smiling. "Just do a test tomorrow morning and we'll play it from there." In those few moments the sex drained out of him and he became a concerned doctor again.

"Dr. Dackel, I have a huge favor to ask. Will you tell me where you're staying in case I need to call you? I promise I won't call unless it's important."

"Sure Carrie," he said caringly. "I'm at the Harmony. Why don't you call me either way and let me know how it turns out."

Suddenly there was a loud bang that sounded like a gunshot coming from the parking lot. Dackel had heard about the tourist shootings in Florida and he instinctively ducked under the table but Carrie just laughed. When he looked up he saw a green van belching blue smoke from its tailpipe and heard it backfire a few more times as it pulled away from just outside the window where they were sitting.

"A little skittish tonight Doc?" giggled Carrie.

"I figured it my wife shooting at me for having coffee with a beautiful girl," he chuckled, his heart still pounding at an almost uncountable rate.

He paid the check, they both got into their own cars and each headed off in a different direction. As he thought about the evening, Dackel became confused. How could Angel, a sexy, sensuous, seductive woman be so easily transformed into Carrie, a scared helpless child? He thought about Carrie the child all the way back to his hotel. Then he got into bed, and thought about Angel the woman while he masturbated.

Chapter 7

At 6:30AM the alarm buzzed. Dackel wasn't even remotely ready to get up. He never should have stayed out so late, he thought to himself. But it certainly was worth it. He jumped into the shower and washed off a mixture of White Linen from the Hispanic girl and Sunflowers from Carrie. He opened the tiny bottle of shampoo thoughtfully supplied by the hotel. He wasn't sure why. He had long ago given up shampoo at home. He had so little hair, it seemed like a waste of money. He liked hotels because they gave you soap and shampoo and usually, a lot of fluffy towels. Not this one. He was somewhat disappointed with the towels at The Harmony. He felt that they were too small and flat and they smelled like the laundry room at the hospital. He would remember to note that on the comment card if he could find one. He always filled out comment cards and always found something negative to write in the hope that he would get a free room or a refund. It often worked. He had four or five certificates for free rooms, unfortunately for places that he would probably never visit again, but, all the same, he treasured them and bragged about them whenever he had the opportunity.

He dressed casually and went down to get the bus to the National Medical Innovations Educational Institute which was located about two miles from the hotel. Most of the other participants were also casually dressed, but the technical advisors were all in perfectly fitting, precisely pressed business suits. When they arrived at the facility, the group was ushered into a casual dining room for the pre-conference continental breakfast. There was orange juice that Dackel recognized as the good stuff, croissants, fruit and of course coffee. One of the young women physicians was complaining that there were no low fat breads or bagels. Dackel was glad. He loved croissants. He loaded his plate with three of them, six pats of butter and a mound of melon, and he went into a corner to eat by himself.

Jerry Evans or Edwards or something like that introduced himself as the president of National Medical Innovations and welcomed everyone to the course. He invited the doctors into the classroom which looked more like a first class airline lounge. The swivel chairs were plush and comfortable. There was a bottle of Perrier at every place along with a leather note pad and a gold (filled) Cross pen. Both were engraved with the doctor's name and the company's.

This company was different. Dackel had been to courses at both Ethicon and U.S. Surgical years ago. They were nice, but nothing like this. He was also curious about all the marketing stuff he was hearing about —the videotape, the media training? He still wasn't sure what it was all about. He still hadn't read the information.

He opened up his information packet and found the syllabus.

SATURDAY

7:00-7:30	Continental Breakfast
7:30-7:45	Introductory Remarks. *Jerry Edmonds, President, National Medical Innovations*
7:45-8:15	Hysterectomy—A Dying Procedure. *Cal Clark, Director of Marketing, National Medical Innovations*
8:15-8:45	The Technique of Endometrial Ablation Using the DAC-III Sonomagnetic Laser- The Beginning of Things to Come. *Mark MacDonald, M.D., Former Professor and Chairman, Department of Obstetrics and Gynecology, Riverside Medical Center, Medical Director, National Medical Innovations*
8:45-9:00	Questions and Answers
9:00-10:00	Marketing Your Practice with the DAC-III Sonomagnetic Laser.

	Beverly DiGioccomo, President, The Marketing Group
10:00-10:30	Coffee Break
10:30-11:15	Insurance Coding and Billing Tips. *Mary Margaret Finney, Former Vice-President Alpha Beta Health Plan, National Medical Innovations Reimbursement Specialist*
11:15-12:00	Introduction to Media Training. *David Evans, Former Anchor WWTT News, Tampa, President, Medical Media*
12:00-2:00	Lunch- Please join us in our VIP Dining Room where our award winning chef will create a meal you won't forget!
2:00-4:00	Lab
4:00	Adjourn. You're on your own to explore Tampa.
	SUNDAY
9:00-10:30	Group A - Video Taping Group B - Lab
10:30-12:00	Group A - Lab Group B - Video Taping
12:00-12:30	Summation and Farewell

Not a bad schedule, but only a 45-minute lecture on how to do the procedure, thought Dackel. It must be as easy as they say it is, and I guess you learn most of it in the lab.

"Okay, let's begin," said Jerry Edmonds. "As you all know, National Medical Innovations is a relatively new company. We have lots of competitors, names you all know. Names like

Stortz, Olympus, ACMI, SLT, Coherent, Hitachi, G.E., Ethicon and BEI just to name a few. Some of them make hysteroscopes, some of them make lasers, some make ultrasound equipment. We make the whole system. It's all integrated into one package. National takes care of every aspect of the endometrial ablation procedure. We manufacture all the hardware, we teach you how to use it and we teach you how to market it. We also teach you how to get reimbursed for it. The bottom line is that it's a win-win-win situation. We win your business, you win a ton of new patients, and your patients win by avoiding hysterectomies. This operation is easy, it's safe as long as you follow a few simple rules, and if you bill it the way we'll teach you, it can be very lucrative.

Edmonds continued with a slide show introducing National Medical Innovations and its products. It was impressive. The television monitors lit up with animation and art that made it hard to nap. Every digital trick in the computer was used. Dackel had always been impressed with those commercials where one face turns into another. Morphing, it was called. That's what they were using here. He watched as a tiny one-room office morphed into a small one story building and ultimately to the twenty story smoked glass building that was now corporate headquarters. He saw the staff of six grow smoothly and magically into a shot of all 750 current employees of National. Edmonds controlled the whole show from a Macintosh G3 Powerbook.

Edmonds told them that most of the computer work had been done by Donny Moline, a young video and computer prodigy. He didn't mention that Donny was watching the virgin voyage of the presentation from a control room in the basement of the building where six remote control cameras with focusing microphones fed him sound and images of the speaker and the participants. He was videotaping the entire session. Later, speakers training consultants would critique the speakers in one-on-one sessions, and the marketing researchers would analyze the reactions of the audience. Moline had even set up some remotely controlled cameras in the hotel and recorded the cocktail party the night before. When it was over, the National staff reviewed the tapes until 2 o'clock in the morning. They were interested in learning what the doctors said to each other about the company, their expectations of the course, and anything else that might help them conduct an efficient and effective workshop. National covered all its bases.

Dackel started to drift but he re-focused in time to hear Edmonds introduce Cal Clark, Director of Marketing for National Medical Innovations.

"The hysterectomy is a dying procedure," shouted Cal with the enthusiasm of a televangelist who had not yet been arrested. "For years, hysterectomy has been the answer to everything." He then proceeded to give a brief history of the hysterectomy, how it was first performed in 1768 in dogs and sheep by Joseph Cavallini. He told how Cavallini concluded that the organ was not essential to life and predicted that in the future it would be possible to pluck the womb "with impunity" from the human body. According to some, that was already happening.

With impressive graphics and animation Clark explained how in 1809 Gotofried Michaelis suggested that combining hysterectomy with amputation of the uterus might ameliorate the hazards of Caesarian Section. Clark showed graphs and pictures that explained how hysterectomies were attempted during the first half of the nineteenth century, but how all the patients died.

He played a computer recreation of Dr. Horatio Robinson Storer of Boston performing one of the first successful hysterectomies in the United States in 1866 and another of the first documented hysterectomy on a woman at the time of a Caesarian section on July 21, 1868. He reminded the class that Dr. Storer was the first surgeon to wear rubber gloves while operating. The graphics were impressive. Somehow, it looked like they had a tape of Storer actually performing a hysterectomy. They all assumed it was Storer. Actually no one in the room had any idea what Storer actually looked like. But nevertheless, the presentation was impressive.

Clark traced the refinement of the procedure through the years and presented statistics showing that by 1975, hysterectomy was the second most commonly performed major operation in the United States, surpassed only by Caesarian Section. Then pausing for dramatic effect, lowering his head, and speaking in almost a whisper, and with a pain and embarrassment in his voice reminiscent of Clinton's "okay, so she blew me" speech, Clark lamented that there were over a half a million hysterectomies done in the United States of America every year. "And the shame of it is," he said, his voice slowly starting to build again, "that most of them are done [the crescendo builds to fortissimo] for excessive bleeding, or fibroids." He finished the sentence exhaustedly with an echoing indignant disdain that he was attempting to convince the audience was coming from deep within the boiler room of his soul.

While all this may have been very interesting, everyone in the room knew it already. Most of it was coming almost word for word from a book called Obstetrics and Gynecology in America, by Harold Speert. The American College of Ob-Gyn had given all of its members a free copy in 1980 and everyone who had ever done any teaching always flipped through it to get the requisite historical background which seemed to preface every lecture.

Continuing in his evangelical style, Clark, who seemed to have found one last pocket of emotional energy, raised the volume and pitch of his voice even higher and exclaimed, once again, that, "In a few years hysterectomy will be taught in medical school from a historical perspective only. Yes doctors, the hysterectomy is a dying procedure, and National Medical Innovations is going to hasten its death, and not a moment too soon!"

Perspiring and spent, Cal left the stage to applause that was polite, but almost insulting considering the effort he had put into his act. Jerry Edmonds then turned the program over to Dr. Mark MacDonald, National's Medical Director. It was a typical flowery introduction complete with the usual expressions like "finest in the country," "extraordinary," "genius," and "fortunate to have him with us."

Dr. MacDonald looked more like a movie star than a medical director. Without going into it, he was what women would call "a hunk," the gay guy who cuts Mrs. Dackel's hair would call "dreamy" and Dackel would admit was "a decent looking guy, if you want to waste your time thinking about things like that."

"Endometrial Ablation with the DAC-III Sonomagnetic Laser is the latest in a string of new technologies that will lead to the demise of the hysterectomy. As you know, several procedures already exist that have decreased the number of hysterectomies performed in the United States and abroad. Myomectomy, or removal of fibroid tumors, is one that I'm sure you are already doing. But as Cal mentioned, many of the hysterectomies performed today are done for excessive bleeding. Once we have ruled out cancer, one of the least invasive surgical techniques for treating excessive bleeding is endometrial ablation or endometrial reduction as some call it.

Traditional endometrial ablation is a procedure in which laser or electrical energy is used to remove or destroy the endometrium, which of course is the innermost lining of the uterus, the part that bleeds. Traditional ablation requires that the surgeon actually drags or rolls the instrument over the entire uterine lining to burn and scar it so it won't bleed anymore.

Balloon endometrial reduction is another technique that makes it a little easier. It follows the same principal of destroying the endometrium, but works a little differently. A balloon is inserted into the uterus and filled with fluid that is heated enough to destroy the cells. Other devices use electrical contacts on the surface of the balloon to supply the energy to destroy the cells. The most elegant and effective system uses low pressure heated saline without the balloon to cook the lining. That one is probably the best of the lot so far, but we're better."

Once again, incredible graphics and illustrations accompanied almost every sentence. The big screen television monitors scattered around the room went from stills, to videos, to live shots of MacDonald.

Still, most of the audience was bored. This was nothing new. Everyone, except Dackel, was already doing one or more of these procedures. Dackel had heard about these techniques, but until today, he had never taken a course to attempt to learn them.

That's why I hired a younger partner, he scowled to himself. I can't be learning all this new shit at my age. I just never should have hired a woman. I knew she couldn't handle full time practice.

"All of these procedures," continued MacDonald, "require a good grasp of the principles of hysteroscopy. It is my understanding that all of the participants in this workshop are experienced hysteroscopists. Is there, by any chance, anyone in the room who is not currently performing hysteroscopy?" Dackel saw no other hands go up and he certainly wasn't about to raise his. Besides he had seen several hysteroscopies on educational videotapes and there was that article in his packet that he would read over during lunch.

"Well this procedure is a no-brainer for an experienced hysteroscopist. All you need to do is position the probe and let the DAC-III do the work. You see, the DAC-III technology combines several of the most advanced technologies into one machine. This is how it works."

"Once the hysteroscope is positioned inside the uterine cavity and the cavity is examined visually, a combination of magnetic, sonar and laser sensors survey the uterus from the inside out. They feed the information into a computer which actually constructs a three dimensional model of the uterus. The computer can differentiate the different types of tissues, so that, for example, the endometrium appears on the screen as a pinkish color. The normal muscle shows up as a dark maroon. The arteries of course are red, the veins blue, and the nerves a light gray. Now if you look at the monitors you'll see the DAC-III's view of a normal uterus."

Suddenly the crowd was hooked. The pictures on the monitors looked as if they were right out of a Netter Atlas. Frank H. Netter, M.D. started out as a successful commercial artist who studied at the National Academy of Design in New York and later at the Art Students' League. But Netter, like many of us, had a mother who wanted to be able to brag to the ladies at the beauty shop about "my son the doctor," so, at her insistence, he went to medical school and by 1933 he completed a residency in surgery at Bellevue Hospital. Although he never practiced clinical medicine, his contributions to the field are well known and greatly appreciated by anyone who ever studied any of the healing arts. Netter was the best and most prolific medical illustrator since da Vinci. He was actually probably better and more prolific than da Vinci, but who's counting. Netter's drawings do what your brain was supposed to have done when you were studying anatomy, they demonstrate relationships. If you studied a Netter drawing it was hard to not understand anatomical relationships.

"And watch this," MacDonald said with an anticipatory smile in his voice. He tickled the touchpad on his Powerbook and the uterus started to rotate clockwise bringing into view the left fallopian tube and the ovary.

He was right. There was a collective "WOW" from the class. Everyone had seen this technology in the MRI lab or the CT room, but never with this much detail and never with such a compact piece of equipment.

"Now, lets look at examples of some uteri with disease. This one has fibroids. You'll notice they show up white. The next is an example of cancer of the endometrium. The computer doesn't want you to miss any cancer so it represents them all in iridescent colors. This particular one is yellow. The next case is cervical cancer. We show that in bright green. And ovarian cancer is this purple color."

"They're not easy to miss, but just in case you do, look in the left upper corner of the screen. You will see the words 'malignancy detected' blinking in red. But here's the best part. By pressing the 'Treat' buttons, the DAC-III will direct a combination of ultrasound, laser light and magnetic energy directly to the abnormal tissue. It knows exactly how to treat each different abnormal tissue with minimal or no damage to the healthy surrounding organs and tissues. It does this by targeting its various energies, in combination, to the specific tissues that you tell it to treat."

"You don't have to aim anything, you don't have to calculate anything. All you need to do is to position the probe and let the DAC-III do the rest. The whole thing takes about 12 minutes.

"The DAC! It's named after me!" Dackel said to the doctor sitting next to him. After the puzzling look, he pointed to his name tag. "See. Dackel. Don't you get it?" This was his first interaction with any of the other participants other than a casual hello. The recipient of what Alfred considered this hilarity smiled politely and fixed his attention back on the speaker.

"At this point, the FDA has only approved the DAC-III for endometrial ablation and if your hospital purchases the system, the computer will be programmed to only perform that procedure, but as we get approval for other procedures we will be able to update your program. For example, you saw how well the fibroid was delineated. We can direct energy to the fibroid and essentially kill it. The body will absorb the dead tissue. And believe me, that's only the beginning. Within a few years, we are confident that the DAC-III will even be able to treat many cancers."

"Those of you who are experienced with performing hysteroscopy under local anesthesia will be happy to know that the DAC-III procedure is no more uncomfortable than a diagnostic hysteroscopy. Because the total time for visual inspection, mapping and treatment can be as long as a half-hour, some of you may want to give your nervous patients a little sedation, but the majority of cases can be performed under local anesthesia. Either way, the patient can leave the hospital the same day."

Alfred Dackel doesn't operate under local anesthesia, he thought to himself. He liked his patients to be asleep and paralyzed. He didn't like it when they moved and he didn't like it when they complained or whimpered. He was also one of the few remaining gynecologists to insist on a complete shave prep of the genital area even though he believed the studies that said that the infection rate was no higher if you didn't shave the patient. He just didn't like having to constantly be moving all that hair out of the way.

"Face it, I'm old fashioned," he would say when his residents or nurses questioned him, "but it's worked for me for a quarter of a century this way and there's no way I'm about to change."

"Here are some 'before' pictures of some diseased animals we treated with the DAC-III. And here are pictures of the same animals three months after treatment," said Dr. MacDonald. The 'after' pictures all looked normal. The fibroids were gone, the cancers were gone, the organs were normal.

"Now I know what you're going to ask," said MacDonald. "Will the tumors re-grow? Will the cancers come back? We don't think so. As you know this technology is new and we've only been testing it in humans for about a year, but our animal studies indicate strongly that once the disease is gone, it's gone. Now obviously, if we're dealing with a cancer that's spread to other parts of the body, this machine won't be much help—yet. But stay tuned. A total body DAC is on the drawing board."

"Now it's time for your questions," MacDonald said, turning up the lights and walking away from his computer and towards his audience.

Everyone had a question. This group, who just a few hours ago was laid back and sleepy was now alive and enthusiastic. They looked like a bunch of fourth graders stretching their hands as high as they could to get chosen to feed the iguana or clap the erasers (in some schools. In others, eraser clapping was a punishment.) They looked like Dackel waving his dollar bills at Angel last night.

An attractive woman in her late forties whose name ended with M.D., Ph.D., J.D., M.B.A. was the first to be called on. Actually, she really didn't wait to be acknowledged. She just started talking as she raised her hand.

"How can you be so sure that this energy will not target healthy cells?"

"We had the same question Dr. Ferrante," answered MacDonald. "We did extensive animal testing with this device and then we used it on the endometria of 10 women who were already scheduled for hysterectomies. We had a team of independent pathologists perform extensive histologic examinations on all of the surrounding tissue and we are now convinced that the DAC-III targets only what we tell it to."

"Dr. Haddad, what can I answer for you?" asked MacDonald as he motioned towards a small Middle Eastern man with a Rolex that would have looked bulky on Arnold Schwartzeneggar.

"We have all been taught that when something seems too good to be true, it usually is. What are the potential complications from this procedure?" asked Haddad, raising his shoulders and turning his palms upward.

"I shared your skepticism for quite a while until I worked with this machine, Doctor," said MacDonald, "and what I have learned is that most of the things that can go wrong are the result of human error. The machine itself has several fail-safes programmed into it, but it is still a machine. The surgeon must be as vigilant during a DAC-III procedure as he or she is during any other operation and, as I stated earlier, the operation should be performed only by experienced hysteroscopists. Any of the complications of hysteroscopy can occur during a DAC-III procedure. Even our sophisticated computer can't prevent a uterine perforation or water intoxication."

"Dr., is it Sha-peer-o or Sha-pie-ro?"

"I'm from New York, it's Sha-pee-ro. I can see what this might be able to do in the future for some of the other diseases you mentioned, but what are the advantages over our traditional methods of endometrial ablation, using electrodes, lasers or heated liquids?"

"Dr. Shapiro," MacDonald answered, "I'm sure that, in your hands, and I'd like to think in mine, endometrial ablation can be safely and effectively carried out by any one of the traditional methods. But this procedure is superior in a number of ways. When you destroy the endometrium with a traditional laser or an electrode, you're essentially destroying the target cell and all the cells surrounding it. It's kind of like napalming a field to get rid of the weeds. The DAC-III doesn't destroy normal tissue. It carefully and precisely kills individual cells. No cells die unless we tell the DAC-III to kill them."

"In addition, this operation is easier. It requires less skill, less time and less anesthesia. It's also safer than the other methods, and when it is approved for procedures other than endometrial ablation, it will offer things that no other procedure offers. Dr. Smith, do you have a question?"

"Yes, I do. You went over the actual mechanics of the procedure rather quickly. I'm not exactly clear on how the DAC-III specifically treats the targeted cells, or in this case, the endometrium."

"Okay, this is as good a time as any to go over some basics," said MacDonald. He had anticipated the question and had a visual presentation already prepared. "Before I get into this I want to reassure you that if you don't follow everything I'm about to tell you, don't worry. You don't really need to understand the theory to learn how to use the machine. The DAC-III utilizes three imaging techniques, ultrasound, magnetic resonance imaging, or MRI, and laser scanning. It is the first system to combine these three techniques to create one image.

You all know about ultrasound. Ultrasound is basically sonar. The ultrasound transducer generates high frequency sound waves that are too high for us to hear. When the sound waves hit something, they bounce back to the machine and create electrical impulses, which get converted to images. Of course the characteristics of whatever they hit determine how fast and hard they bounce back. Like if you throw a ball against a wall it bounces back fast and hard. If you throw it against a pillow, the pillow absorbs the energy and it doesn't bounce back as fast or as far. So, different reflected sound waves from different kinds of tissues create different patterns of electrical energy and result in unique images for each tissue."

Dackel listened and understood what MacDonald was saying and he tried to pay attention to what he said next, but the metaphor about throwing the ball against the wall took control of his mind and pulled it back to the alley next to Red's house where the boys played a variety of games, most of which required throwing a ball against a wall. He shook his head to get rid of the image so he could pay attention to the speaker. As he shook it, MacDonald happened to look up.

"You disagree, doctor?"

“No, no,” said Dackel, embarrassed and blushing, “just, heh heh, trying to shake some water out of my ears from my shower this morning.” Why did I say that, he said to himself, that was really stupid.

“I guess that happens to all of us occasionally,” said MacDonald. “Well, anyway, that’s the basic explanation of ultrasound, but the diagnostic ultrasound component of the DAC-III is more sophisticated than the ones you’re used to. It allows us to get microresolution images of these tissues so that we can clearly differentiate normal from abnormal tissues. But even with microresolution, the problem is that ultrasound is only good for visualizing some tissues. It’s not that great for others, so that’s why we add to the ultrasound information additional data gathered by MRI or magnetic resonance imaging.

I know we all order MR’s on our patients, but I, for one, wasn’t exactly sure how MR worked until I started working with the DAC-III, so I’ll give you all a short course right now.

All matter is made up of atoms. Atoms are basically protons surrounded by orbiting electrons. There are also neutrons in atoms, but we don’t need to worry about them for the moment. Magnetism is a property of all matter. It results from the orbiting of the electrons around the protons in the atoms. The movement of these electrons result in what physicists call angular momentum or ‘spin’. This creates a magnetic field around the proton. Got that?”

All heads, even Dackel’s nodded affirmatively.

“Okay, let’s go on. Protons in a magnetic field behave like children’s tops that spin around and wiggle and wobble. The rate of the wobbling, which we call precession is the ‘resonance’ part of magnetic resonance imaging. Now, all of the tissues in the body contain hydrogen atoms. Normally the protons in these hydrogen atoms point randomly in different directions, but when you expose these protons to a powerful magnetic field, created by the MRI machine, they line up parallel to each other.”

Dackel was now officially lost in the woods and hoping that MacDonald’s next sentence would clear things up.

“And here comes the confusing part. If you then hit these lined up hydrogen atom protons with a strong burst of radio waves, it knocks the protons out of alignment. When the burst stops, they fall back into alignment and as they do, they produce a detectable radio signal. Magnetic coils in the MRI machine take these signals and convert them into an image.”

Dackel's wish did not come true but everyone else seemed to be following and MacDonald continued.

"Different tissues contain different amounts of hydrogen so they send different strength signals which create different images. For example, fat contains a lot of hydrogen, so on an MRI, fat produces a bright image. Bone has very little hydrogen so bone appears black."

Dackel was tempted to raise his hand and ask why don't they make it so that bone is white, but he decided against it.

"The DAC-III is also capable of the latest variation of MRI, called MRS, magnetic resonance spectroscopy. It makes the MR even more sensitive. It was first used in brain imaging, but we have adapted it to the pelvis. The way it works is pretty easy to understand. Most diseased tissue behaves differently than normal tissue. It undergoes different chemical reactions and therefore creates different metabolites or chemical products of the reactions. The patterns of these chemicals are distinct enough to create a 'biochemical fingerprint.' The DAC-III is programmed to recognize these patterns and diagnose many diseases without requiring a biopsy or tissue sample. Is everybody still with me?"

Dackel watched as all the other heads in the room nodded affirmatively. He just sighed and closed his eyes for a few seconds, the same few seconds that MacDonald happened to look at him.

"Are you okay doctor?"

"Dackel suddenly opened his eyes and tried to find something to say, but nothing would come out so he just nodded.

"Now, here's the neat part. In the past, in order to do an MRI, the patient's whole body had to be slid into a large cylinder. The beauty and uniqueness of the DAC-III, and there are so many beauties and uniquenesses, is that we have figured out how to emulate a magnetic field that we can deliver through a hysteroscope."

The room was silent, with every last attention neuron focused on the speaker. They had just learned the secret that National had been keeping for the last five years, the technology that would, no doubt, make it the most successful company of its kind. But MacDonald had even more to tell them.

"The laser scanner adds to the image by creating a topographic map of the tissues. I won't insult you by lecturing you on laser physics, but you all know that a laser at low power can scan without damage, like the bar code reader in the supermarket, or like this pointer I'm using. When the DAC-III shifts into the treatment phase, however, the laser's power and wavelength are increased so that it can destroy the target tissue.

Anyway, we'll talk about treatment in a few minutes. Back to establishing the target. The computer integrates the images of the ultrasound, the MRI and the laser scanner and creates a three dimensional model of the pelvis.

Once the computer creates the model of the pelvis, it analyzes the various tissues that comprise it. We have taught the DAC-III the difference between endometrial tissue and the underlying muscle. We have also taught it the difference between benign and malignant endometrium. We are in the process of teaching it to recognize malignant ovarian tissue. We hope that it will be able to detect a nest of as few as ten malignant cells."

The audience would have become even more silent if such a thing had been possible. The doctors, even Dackel, were in absolute awe of this machine and what it could do.

"Okay, now the good part. To answer your question, Dr. Smith, the DAC-III..."

"Excuse me, interrupted Dackel, "I forgot Dr. Smith's question. Could you repeat it?" He was so caught up in the excitement, he didn't even realize that he asked the question until it was half out.

"Sure, Dr. Dackel, Dr. Smith wanted to know how the DAC-III specifically treats the targeted cells."

"Oh, that's right, I'm sorry," said Dackel, realizing that once again, he sounded kind of dumb.

"Once the DAC-III constructs a three dimensional computerized map or model, it digitally marks the boundaries of the area to be treated. The magnetic field holds the protons in their lined up position and identifies the target cells. Then it directs a combination of laser or light energy, and ultrasonic vibration directly and specifically to the targeted cells. Neither the laser nor the ultrasonic energy generated by the DAC-III is destructive by itself. Only when they both hit the same tissue at the same time will they destroy it. Since these energies travel at different wavelengths, the computer is able to send each independently and safely through the normal tissues. The only place that they intersect is at the target tissue. Normal tissues are spared.

I hope I'm not losing anyone. Let me do a quick review. We have a tissue we want to destroy. We don't want to destroy any of the normal surrounding tissue. The DAC-III targets the specific tissue that we want to get rid of. It lines up the atoms of the tissue with magnetism and then sends out two different kinds of energy that are harmless until they meet. They meet at the target tissue and destroy it. Got it?"

The room collectively nodded.

"I have to remind you again that this technology is only in its infancy. We chose endometrial ablation because it was the easiest model to test. In the near future we expect to be able to expand its use to the gastrointestinal tract, the circulatory system and eventually the brain."

"And up till now, we have only treated benign disease states in humans, but we feel, and our animal studies bear this out, that the DAC-III will act even more effectively on malignant tissue. It's easy to identify and should be easy to treat. Dr. Dackel do you have a question?"

"Yes, I understand how the laser can destroy tissue, but how does the ultrasound work? Why doesn't diagnostic ultrasound destroy cells? We use it for looking at fetuses. They aren't affected at all."

"At high frequencies, ultrasound is used for diagnostic imaging. Lower frequencies are the ones that do the damage. The best way to understand it is to remember that sound creates pressure waves, which transfer energy to whatever they contact. Think about listening to your stereo. You can hear the high frequencies, but when you turn up the low frequency bass, you can actually feel the sound through your body. Now your stereo puts out a whole different range of frequencies than an ultrasound generator, but the principle's the same. And if the frequency is just right, a very interesting phenomenon can occur. It's called cavitation."

"If you hit a cell with the right frequency of ultrasound, gas and vapor bubbles or cavities form and then collapse in the liquid components of the cell. When the bubbles collapse, major chemical changes in the cell can result that can destroy the cell. Does that answer your question Dr. Dackel?"

"It does, thank you," he said. Of course while he was saying it, he was thinking that he had no fucking idea what the guy was talking about.

"I have one other question," said Dackel. "What does DAC-III stand for?"

"I'm sorry," said MacDonald, "I should have mentioned that at the beginning. D, A, and C were the first letters of the last names of the three biomedical engineers who built the machine, but now we say it stands for Diagnose And Cure. The III represents the three technologies that combine to make it work, laser, MR and Ultrasound. I'm sure that some of you have more questions, however, my time is up. But don't worry, most of them will be answered by the end of the lab today.

The next speaker was introduced as Beverly DiGioccomo, President of The Marketing Group. She was what Dackel's mother Dora would have called a "smart looking woman." She was thirty something, tall and slender with shiny, rich chestnut hair—smooth hair—rich lady's hair—television anchor hair as his father would have called it. She wore the obligate blue suit and white silk blouse, but her heels were a bit higher than typical corporate, and her skirt a bit shorter. He wondered if she was wearing pantyhose or stockings. And if they were stockings, were they the ones with the elastic on the top or the garter kind. And what about her panties? Dackel guessed that she wore expensive, very lacy French-cut fleshtones, nothing overtly sleazy or whorey, and definitely not a thong.

He had become quite good at guessing what kind of undergarments his patients wore. Some of them stuffed them into their purses or hid them under a pile of clothes in the examining room, but not all of them did. It was interesting to him that in the office, guess the underwear was just a game he played when he was bored. In the office, underwear had absolutely no sexual overtones (undertones?), but when he took of his white coat, he became a guy again. He wished that just once, he could look at a woman on the street or in a social situation without thinking about her underwear or how she was shaved or whether he could get her or what she would be like in bed. He knew it wasn't right, he just couldn't help it.

Occasionally he would feel like a pervert when he played his underwear game, but compared with what other doctors did, this was nothing. He read in the paper that a family physician had installed a peephole in his examining rooms so he could watch his patients change. A pediatrician friend of his bragged that he had slept with more than thirty-five mothers of his patients. "Why else would I make housecalls?" he joked.

Beverly DiGioccomo didn't speak from the podium. She walked through the audience while she talked, like a television talk show host. When she asked a rhetorical question or made a point, she picked one person to look at, and she looked at that person right in the eyes.

Dackel wasn't really concentrating on what she was saying at first, but he knew she was good. Finally he was able to focus on the content of her lecture.

"...so given all that, it certainly makes sense to do some kind of marketing, especially when you have an innovation like the DAC-III to offer," she said staring directly into Dackel's eyes. "I know that some of you think that marketing is tacky, and if it isn't done right, I agree with you, but what we're going to talk about today is nothing but high road, high line, class marketing. What you're going to sell is an image—an image of a caring, competent physician who goes out of her or his way to offer the most up to date, safe, medically sound treatments. And isn't that accurate?" she said, now locking eyes with Dr. Shapiro who was nodding his head ever so slightly, but nonetheless, affirmatively.

Beverly DiGioccomo spent the next ten minutes giving examples of her previous successes like how, with a few well placed news stories, she created the Tickle Me Elmo craze of Christmas 1996, and how she convinced a generation of yuppies that Vietnamese pot bellied pigs made good pets and that suspenders were chic.

She then explained how to use radio, television and newspapers to generate free publicity. Metzger-Minkman had said the same thing. She explained how giving talks at local schools and churches can lead to referrals. She even explained how consumer advocacy groups, even the crazy ones, can be your friends. Dackel wasn't sure about these groups. One, called SHE, Stop Hysterectomy Exploitation, had once picketed his home because they found out that he had done more hysterectomies that year than anyone in his hospital. He called the cops and had them arrested but not until after he turned on his lawn sprinkler.

DiGioccomo distributed a spiral bound booklet with reprints of her articles from Medical Economics and Forbes. The last page was a list of other marketing consultants around the country with whom she had worked and felt comfortable recommending. Sure enough, listed in the Mid-Atlantic States region was none other than Deborah Metzger-Minkman who was not, by the way, the only hyphenated name on the list.

The coffee break was next. Everyone took off for the bathrooms and then to the refreshments. It was the usual, leftover croissants and fruit from breakfast, chocolate chip cookies, coffee and soft drinks.

"Good course," Dackel said to a man who looked to be about his age.

"Sounds impressive," he replied, "but they don't seem to be spending a lot of time on the medicine part. I would like to see some clinical studies, some pathology slides, and some of the animal work. I don't see where they're going to have time to get into that."

"Yep," said Dackel, walking back to his seat feeling embarrassed that he hadn't even thought about those aspects.

"I really am a loser," he said to himself.

Mary Margaret Finney was next. She was so non-descript looking that he didn't even make the effort to evaluate her appearance. He did guess that she had bad breath, and had he gotten within five feet of her, he would have congratulated himself on the call. After distributing a booklet on reimbursement tips and strategies, she explained that DAC-III Sonomagnetic Laser Endometrial ablation was a new procedure that would not be immediately recognized by the insurance companies.

"They're very slow to cover new operations for a lot of reasons. First, they want to make sure the operation works. They don't want to pay for you to do research. They also want to be sure that there are no less expensive alternatives. If there are, then we have a fight. That will be the case with the DAC-III if we're not careful. We won't have to convince the carriers that this is cheaper than a hysterectomy, but we will have to show the advantages over traditional endometrial ablations, which, by the way, many carriers don't even pay for yet."

She then went through a number of things that could be done until the company starts to pay for the procedure. She explained how to bend the codes to the point that they were ready to snap.

"You can bill for a hysteroscopy. They'll pay for that. If you're lucky, you'll find a little polyp or a small fibroid that you can pluck out before you start the endometrial ablation. If you do, you can bill for a polypectomy or removal of the fibroid or myoma, which is coded as hysteroscopic myomectomy. Of course you all know that the reimbursement for a hysteroscopic myomectomy is more than for a polypectomy, and sometimes you can't tell the difference between a firm polyp and a mushy fibroid, if you get my drift."

She had some really good ideas that Dackel hoped he would remember, not only about the DAC-III procedure, but about billing in general. But he knew that he probably wouldn't remember any of them. He started to drift again, thinking about Carrie and Metzger-Minkman. He even spent a little more time on Beverly DiGioccomo's underwear.

Media training with Dave Evans was next. Media training. Who ever thought I would be taking a course in media training, Dackel said to himself. He was aware, though, that more and more television and radio stations had doctors on the news or doing talk shows. It all started with Dr. Art Ulene, "America's family doctor." Dackel used to watch him on the "Today Show." He was always impressed with his manner and presence, but mostly by the information he dispensed. It was always accurate, understandable and important. He remembered several instances when a patient of his heard something on the "Today Show" about blood in the stool or lumps under the arm or whatever, and came to see him in the office. Dackel figured that over the years, in his practice alone, Dr. Art Ulene had saved a dozen lives.

Dr. Timothy Johnson was another one. He started out on "Good Morning America," and before you knew it he was on the "ABC News" and even "20/20." He thought Johnson was a very smart, responsible and levelheaded doctor, but there was a time that he pissed him off. A few years ago "20/20" did a story on hysteroscopy, how it was superior to plain D&C's and how it wasn't being done enough. Dackel didn't see the piece, but he was questioned by almost every patient he scheduled for a D&C. He would blow them off telling them that you can't believe everything you see on TV and how Tim Johnson was not even a gynecologist.

Ten years later and I'm finally learning hysteroscopy, he said to himself. Then he admitted, for the first time, that all along he knew 20/20 was right and that he had always respected Tim Johnson as both a doctor and a communicator.

Dave Evans took the podium.

"Doctors don't do well on television and radio. The reason for that is that they don't teach you how to do it in medical school. Remember, when you go into a studio, you're on someone else's turf. There are wires and lights and people rushing around. There are machines and dials and meters that are strange to you. You are the stranger. You are the visitor. You are not in control, and you are not used to that. If I would walk into your operating room I'd feel the same way.

But doctors are quick learners, and in the next forty-five minutes, I'm going to teach you everything you need to know about being a guest on a television or radio show. I want to start out by showing you how not to be. I want you to watch a segment from an old Bob Newhart show when he was invited to be a guest on an early morning television interview show. In this show you'll see every mistake you can make." He started the tape and almost instantly, Dackel remembered the show. He was a big Newhart fan.

"Now let's talk about Dr. Hartley's appearance," said Evans while a few of the doctors were still laughing. "First off, he immediately lost control of the interview. He wanted to talk about psychology. She went directly to fees. He let her set the agenda, probably because he had none. You saw how the host fished around until she led him into a trap. What I want you to remember is that when you go on one of these shows you are there for one reason—to promote the DAC-III procedure. To do that you'll have to look good, you'll have to know what you want to say and you'll have know how to say it. If the host doesn't give you an opportunity to say what you came to say, you'll have to make your own opportunity."

Evans went to the blackboard. Interesting, he was the one lecturing about the electronic media, and he was the only one who didn't use hi-tech slides and graphics. He used the blackboard.

"There are three techniques that you must learn if you want to be an effective guest, and I mean effective from your standpoint, not the host's. First, you must learn how to 'fire the cannon.'" He took a piece of chalk and wrote F the C.

Dackel chuckled out loud. Apparently he was the only one in the room who looked at F the C and thought of something dirty.

"By that I mean state the message you came to state. In this case, it's that you can offer a new, state of the art alternative to hysterectomy. You want to get that in at least three times during the interview. Nothing else you say is as important as your cannonball."

"The next thing you have to be able to do is get to a point where you can fire the cannon effectively. This can be difficult to do if your host has another agenda. Sometimes the host hasn't prepared for you and doesn't have any idea what you're there to talk about. And sometimes, the interviewers are just plain dumb. But it's your job to get into position to 'fire the cannon.'"

"One of the techniques you can use is called the 'bridge.' You see politicians doing this all the time. Bob Dole bridged all the time, but usually very clumsily, and some say that it cost him votes. A reporter would ask him a question about why he voted for or against a particular issue when he was a senator. He would answer something like, 'How I voted isn't the issue, the issue is that the tax and spend Democrats...'"

"Do you see what I mean? He didn't address the issue, he just bridged over to line up his cannon. If you don't want to be ineffective and obnoxious as he was, you can always answer the question and then go for the bridge. For example, suppose the host asks a question like, 'Doctor, isn't it true that some surgeons are performing new operations that they're really not trained to do?'" Dackel listened closely to this one.

"You might answer, 'Yes Mr. Koppel, that can potentially happen and our medical associations and credentialing committees are working very hard to make sure that a doctor is well trained before he or she attempts any new procedure, but it is also important to realize that some of these new operations such as the DAC-III procedure are easy to learn and may save more than 200,000 women a year from hysterectomies.'"

"Did you see the bridge?" asked Evans, "Wasn't it smooth?"

Everyone in the room seemed interested in what Evans was saying. Dackel was trying to figure out why he kept busting on Bob Dole. But you could even see Dackel's wheels start to turn when he gave the next example.

"How would you handle this one," he asked. "Suppose the interviewer said something like, 'I think you doctors charge way too much.' How would you respond to that? Dr. Haddad?"

"I would explain," said Haddad, "that what we bill has not a thing to do with what we are actually reimbursed by managed care, and that our expenses such as malpractice insurance continue to go up every year while our reimbursements are going down."

"That's an honest answer, Doctor, but not the one I would like to see you give. Remember, you're not there to talk about reimbursements or managed care or malpractice insurance. You're there to what? Group?"

"Fire the cannon," replied everyone not even remotely in unison.

"Okay, so let's figure out a way to line up the cannon. I would suggest a technique called 'the hook.' You hook your interviewer into asking the right question. So to the question about charging too much, I would respond, 'Yes, Sally Jesse, [a snicker from the audience] fees are an important and controversial issue, but I think that they are only the second most important issue here.' Now any half decent host is going to immediately ask the obvious question, which is?"

"What's the first?" answered the entire class in a manner much closer to unison.

"Aha," said Evans. "See, you couldn't resist. I hooked you!"

He went through several more examples and then did a few role plays. Dackel volunteered to be a guest on a mock Geraldo show. As soon as he finished, Evans realized another issue needed to be addressed. Trying not to be obvious, he said, "Before we go on, this would be a good time to talk about appearance. If you're going to do TV you need to follow some rules. Dr. Dackel, you look very relaxed in that chair, but it's not right for television. I'd like you to sit up straight and lean forward a little. It gives the impression that you have something important to say if you sit forward in your chair."

Dackel, a little embarrassed, sat up and leaned forward forcing his knees apart even more than they had been in Scampers the night before. His hands hung between his thighs.

"Doctor, I'm going to teach you the executive pose," said Evans. "Cross your legs at the knee with the crossed leg pointing toward your interviewer. If you cross away from the interviewer you give the impression of being afraid of him. Rest you hands on your lap, one on top of the other. Uh- a little closer to your knees, Doctor, we don't want anyone to get the wrong impression." The room snickered. "That's good, but don't interlock your fingers. When you do that it keeps you from using your hands to gesture when you're trying to make a point. Now, you watch the next time the president or some CEO is interviewed. If they're sitting, I'll bet you this is how they'll be sitting."

Evans continued with a few more rules: "Wear over-the-calf socks; wear a powder blue or gray shirt because white is too bright for the camera; wear a dark suit; never wear anything with checks; don't wear jangly jewelry; make sure your zipper's up."

"Remember, this is just an introductory session. I would suggest that if you are planning to do any TV or radio, that you find someone in your area to spend a few hours coaching you. If you look in the packet I handed out you'll see, in the very back, a list of media trainers who I think are very good."

Dackel glanced at the list. Sure enough, there it was, taking up much more space than it should have—Deborah Metzger-Minkman.

Chapter 8

Lunch was every bit as spectacular as everything else that National Medical Innovations provided. The dining room was paneled with deep cherry wood. The tableware was as fine as he'd seen in any restaurant, and at each place was a menu embossed in gold leaf with the doctor's name.

Dackel opened his menu. Printed above the list of courses was a note that read,

> Welcome to the National Medical Innovations Dining Room, Dr. Dackel. This afternoon you will be treated to a gourmet lunch prepared by Jonathan Michael, a graduate of the Culinary Institute of America. In keeping with your request for a low fat meal, your choices have all been adapted to contain less than two grams of fat per course. We hope you enjoy your lunch.

Low fat! He yelled (to himself), damn that woman.

He didn't even know whom he was damning. It could have been either his wife or his secretary. Probably someone called to see if he had any dietary restrictions and one or the other of them told them that he was on a low fat diet. Now what was he going to do, make a scene and ask for another menu or just bite the high fiber bullet? Although it was out of character for him, he chose the latter.

He wound up choosing black bean soup, mixed greens with fat-free raspberry vinaigrette, no fat vegetable risotto and, for dessert, fresh fruit. He sat next to a National salesman he hadn't yet met, and a young Asian woman physician who he sat next to on the bus that morning, but didn't remember. He was, of course, embarrassed when he introduced himself again and she said,

"Yes, we've already met."

He put the other foot in his mouth when he said,

"Oh, I'm sorry, I thought I met the other Chinese girl."

"I'm Korean and I haven't been a girl for twenty-five years," she said, seriously at first, but when she saw his puzzled look, she broke out in a laugh. He laughed too, but he wasn't sure why.

"What do you think so far?" he asked her.

"I think this procedure sounds like it has a lot of promise, but I felt that way about other devices and procedures that turned out to be flashes in the pan. I remember when I was a resident, everyone was saying that the laser was the best way to treat cervical dysplasia. We were using cryosurgery to freeze them at that time and we were happy with it. The practice that I eventually went into even bought its own laser. It was used, but it was still $40,000. Well, you know what happened to lasers. Electrosurgery with the loop electrodes came out a few years later, and I haven't fired up my laser since. Then as soon as we spent four grand for an electrosurgical generator, the bipolar system came out and the one we had became obsolete.

Dackel was still treating cervical dysplasia by freezing the cervix, in fact, he had just started. The only reason he finally gave in was that his managed care carriers were not approving cold knife cone biopsies for most of his patients with abnormal Pap smears. Cold knife referred to a regular scalpel. In the past, if one of Dackel's patients had an abnormal Pap smear, and the biopsy concurred that it needed to be treated, he would admit her to the hospital, shave her of course, put her to sleep and actually cut a cone shaped hunk of tissue from her cervix. Cold knife cone biopsies are significantly bloodier than the newer methods, they require hospitalization and anesthesia and post-operative bleeding occurs frequently. Cold cones are still indicated in some circumstances, but not nearly as often as they were twenty years ago.

Laser and the electrosurgical loop treatments are done with local anesthesia and can be performed in the office. The laser vaporizes the tissue. The loop shaves it out. Cryosurgery is a procedure that freezes the cervix in two minutes, in the office and without anesthesia. Over the next few weeks, the frozen tissue dies and is absorbed by the body. Once Dackel tried cryosurgery, he was very happy with it.

Why am I so slow to try new things? he often asked himself. He never got an answer.

His bean soup was served. It was delicious, but when he glanced over at Dr. Kim's cream of carrot soup, he once again cursed both his wife and his secretary (because he still wasn't sure which one to curse.) The salad was a salad. The vinaigrette was okay, nothing like the blue cheese that teased him as it slowly plopped from the ladle onto Dr. Kim's croutons.

"Dr. Dackel, haven't had a chance to introduce myself." said the National salesman to his right. "Bill Horn with National Medical."

Stepford children, Dackel thought. If the Stepford wives ever had children they would all look like this and they would all become salesmen.

"Hello Bill," said Dackel. "Nice diggs you guys have."

"I'm glad you're enjoying yourself," Horn replied.

Who said anything about enjoying myself, Dackel thought, but then he had to admit he was enjoying himself. For the first time in a long time, he felt good about himself and, more importantly, he was once again becoming excited about medicine.

"Doctor," Bill spoke in a hushed voice so that Dr. Kim couldn't hear, "a few of us are going over to a gentleman's club tonight, and I was wondering whether you might like to join us."

It was not unusual for "the boys" to get together for activities of that sort during conventions and meetings. The salesmen could usually be counted on to find the best places and to foot the bill.

"Gentleman's club?" asked Dackel playing dumb, "I'm not sure I know what a gentleman's club is," he replied, just to see how Mr. Perfect was going to communicate the concept of a titty bar while trying not to offend him, just in case he was the kind to be offended by the invitation.

What he didn't know is that while reviewing the tape of the cocktail party, the National staff all saw that the camera happened to record Dackel looking at a piece of paper which he took out of his pocket as he was leaving. As the camera zoomed in, the whole staff laughed as they watched him double-check the address for Scampers.

"Well some of them are very well run, high class restaurants and bars with Las Vegas style go-go dancers. Why don't you look at some of the ads in the phone book and get a better idea of what they're about before you decide whether you'd like to join us."

This guy is smooth, thought Dackel.

"I'll let you know," he said.

"What are you two boys whispering about," asked a large densely built woman in her fifties with big brassy blond hair that could be kindly described as ratty, and a cigarette and whiskey voice. "My name's Mary McLeod. I'm Professor and Chairperson at University General in Brooklyn. You wouldn't be talking about the adult entertainment I've been hearing so much about down here, would you?" she asked, the last few words turning into a laugh that turned into a wheeze, then a cough and then terminated in what sounded like a death gurgle.

Dackel looked to Horn hoping he would be able to come up with the right words. He surprised him by looking directly at her and saying,

"Sure are Doc, want to join us?"

Everyone at the table laughed, but before the conversation went any further, the waiters came with the main course.

Dackel's main course was actually very good but when he saw Horn's lobster Newburg and Kim's chicken with grapes in cream sauce, he wanted to just reach over and steal a bite. Dessert was even more frustrating. He was served a nice assortment of berries. Horn got a creme brulee and Kim made orgasm sounds with every bite of her warm chocolate cake with bittersweet chocolate icing. He broke down and called the waiter over.

"Can you get me one of those?" he asked pointing at the last bite of Dr. Kim's gustatory aphrodisiac.

"Certainly Doctor," said the waiter returning shortly with yet another layer of sludge for Dackel's coronary arteries.

After lunch almost everyone went to make calls. This is standard at most out of town medical meetings and there's usually a line at the three or four payphones that are normally available. National Medical Innovations must have taken that into consideration when they built their facility because just off the dining room was a communications room with thirty individual booths, actually small carrels, each with a telephone, a fax machine and a Pentium computer with a modem. Dackel called Arlene. She wasn't home. Saturday, one o'clock, she was probably getting her hair done or her feet scraped or hot wax poured over her body, or something. He left a message.

"Hi, I'm at the meeting, things are going okay. Talk to you later." After he hung up, he felt a little guilty, not about going to the strip club last night, but about the cup of coffee that followed.

He called the office of the practice that was covering for him.

"Woman's Health Associates answering service, would you mind holding?" and before he was able to say that yes he would mind, he heard Kenny G. music. He hated Kenny G. He thought his music was whiny. The longer he held, the more he hated Kenny G. and the more he hated answering services. Dackel was fanatical about returning phone calls. He had been through three services in the last year and a half. He fired the first one because he found a cheaper one, but the cheap one was terrible. He sometimes got his messages an hour after the patient called, so he fired them after a month and went to a new one which promised that they would pick up by the third ring and guaranteed that if you were unhappy with the service, you would not be charged for the week. He hadn't paid a dime since signing on with them.

After four or five minutes an attendant got on.

"Answering service, can I help you?"

"Yes, I'm Dr. Dackel. Women's Health is covering me this weekend and I'd like to know whether any of my patients have called."

"I'm sorry, we don't have a Dr. Dackel on our service."

"I know you don't," he sighed, "I'm Dr. Dackel. I need to speak to the doctor on call from Women's Health."

"Is this in reference to a particular patient?"

"Listen to me, you moron," yelled Dackel. "Who is on call for the practice?

"That would be Dr. Porter."

"Where can I find him?"

"Hold please."

He was forced to listen to another three minutes of Kenny G. before another voice returned.

"Women's Health answering service, can you hold?"

This time he caught her before she put him on hold.

"No I can't hold! I've been holding! This is Dr. Dackel and I need to speak to the doctor on call for Women's Health."

"Hold please."

He gave up and slammed the phone down.

"Screw it."

He knew he didn't have to worry. Women's Health Associates was a group of six superb physicians. They were all university trained, bright, aggressive and highly competent doctors. He trusted them enough to send his wife to them for her gynecologic care.

He made one more call, this one to the hotel to check for messages. He didn't really expect any, but he was kind of hoping that there would be one there from Carrie. There was. She left a number for him to call before 1:00. It was now 1:25. He tried the number but there was no answer and no machine.

He tried to tell himself that he was excited that she called because he was curious about her pregnancy test, but he couldn't deny the definite twitch that he felt when he got the message.

Chapter 9

An attractive woman in a powder blue scrub suit escorted the group into the lab. She introduced herself as Loretta Conklin.

"Welcome to National Medical's state of the art Virtual Endoscopic Surgery Learning Facility.

Endoscopic surgery is any operation done through a telescope of some kind. Sometimes the telescope can be passed directly into the body through an existing opening, down the throat, through the nose, through the anus, through the urethra, or through the vagina and cervix. Sometimes an incision must be made, usually a small (half inch) incision. There is often a camera attached to the telescope to transmit the picture to a television. Other small instruments such as scissors, lasers, and graspers can also be passed into the body. The advantages of endoscopic surgery are that it is usually performed in an outpatient setting, there is less blood loss and the patient heals much more quickly. In addition, most of the pain following surgery is a result of the incisions into the body, not the work that is done once the surgeon gets in and endoscopic incisions are usually much smaller than the kind you need for traditional surgery.

I think you'll find this afternoon's experience will be both fun and educational," said Loretta. "You'll notice that each of you has your own virtual operating suite, and as the afternoon progresses we'll teach you how to take advantage of the most hi-tech learning that you have ever experienced.

First, a little about our surgical education capabilities. There are two different types of computer assisted surgery that this lab is equipped to demonstrate. You will be experiencing both this afternoon. The first is virtual or computer generated surgery. This technology has existed for a few years, but the problem has been to make the images realistic, and to make the tissue resistance accurate.

As you know, it feels different when you're cutting different tissues. Even if you just push on tissue with an instrument, we felt that you should be able to feel that tissue push in or deform. The Visible Human Project from the National Library of Medicine has made it possible to construct accurate, lifelike three-dimensional images, and the tissue resistance or deformation problem has been solved by a software package called TELEOS.

The hardware that we use consists of two scissor grip instrument handles that are hooked up to a sensor that feeds into an optical encoder and ultimately interfaces with the simulation program. The software can make those handles anything we want, scissors, graspers, whatever.

What the engineers here at National Medical Innovations have been able to do is integrate the TELEOS program with three-dimensional real time images creating a realistic looking, realistic feeling surgical learning model.

The other kind of surgery you will experience this afternoon is what is called robotic or remote control surgery. Although it won't be used for endometrial ablation, it has many other uses and I'd like to demonstrate it for you.

Since endoscopic procedures usually require very little hand to tissue contact, it is perfect for robotic surgery. Let me give you an example. If you are operating with a scissors, you're not touching the blades, you are actually just manipulating the handle at the end of a long thin shaft. When you open the handles, the movement is mechanically transferred to the blades and the blades open. When you close the handles, the blades cut the tissue.

Now suppose that instead of the movements of the handle being transferred mechanically, they are transmitted electronically to a robotically controlled scissors. The blades of that scissors will still respond to your movement of the handles. You don't need to be in the same room as your patient. You don't even need to be on the same planet."

"What's the practical application of this technology?" asked someone who hadn't asked any questions up to now.

"Well, suppose a family physician in a remote area has a case that he can't handle by himself. He could insert the instruments, hook up the robotic arms and dial in to one of you who could complete the surgery.

Actually, the military has played a big part in developing this technology and I think it's easy to see how they might use it. There has also been a great deal of interest from NASA. With a minimum of training, an astronaut could be trained to set up the robot, and someone in Houston, or anywhere else, could do the first appendectomy on the moon."

Loretta then took a piece of raw chicken breast and placed it in the center of an operating table under an array of robotic arms. One arm held a telescope, another was attached to a grasping forceps and another to a scissors. She walked to the other side of the stage where there was an identical set of instruments. Connected to each instrument was a wire.

She looked into the television monitor and saw the chicken breast and the robotic forceps and scissors. Ms. Conklin manipulated her telescope. The telescope above the chicken breast moved. The picture on the monitor reflected the change in position of the scope. While looking at the monitor, she moved her graspers towards the image of the chicken. The robotic graspers moved toward the chicken. She opened the jaws of her graspers. The jaws of the robotic graspers opened, and when she closed them on the chicken, the robot mimicked her. She then moved her scissors toward the specimen and by remote control, she cut off a small piece of skin.

Everyone was impressed. Dackel felt overwhelmed. He was sure he didn't have the eye-hand coordination for this, but then again, this technology would probably not be in general use until long after he retired.

"Now, let's go into the next room so you can play too."

The room was large with twenty operating tables surrounding a central elevated stage. On each table was a mannequin covered with a surgical drape. There was what appeared to be a complete set of surgical instruments that had wires leading from them to a large harness connected to a computer. There were two television monitors positioned just as they would be in a real operating room.

"Doctors, these operating rooms are set up just like the ones you work in every day," said Loretta, "and we have supplied a virtual patient for each of you to learn on."

Most surgical technique courses use animals in their "wet labs." Thousands of pigs, dogs and goats give up their lives every year so that doctors can make their mistakes on something that can't sue them. It presents a real dilemma for most surgeons. Most of them fully understand the importance of the use of animals in medical research and education, but few, even the hunters, do not feel bad when they are the ones directly responsible for the death of any living creature in the lab.

"National has set up this virtual reality lab to demonstrate the use of the DAC-III system, but first, we want you to become familiar with virtual surgery, so we set up several tasks for you to master before we go on to the DAC-III Sonomagnetic Laser Endometrial Ablation technique. Each of you will have a surgical assistant to work with. None of them are physicians, but they all are very familiar with the equipment and they're pretty darn good at performing the tasks.

The sales reps then scattered, each going to a different table.

John Duke was Dackel's surgical assistant. He was wearing a crisply starched scrub suit with his name and National's logo on the pocket.

"Hi, Dr. Dackel," he smiled, "ready to boogie."

"Ready to boogie?" Dackel thought. "Ready to boogie?" He was going to say something sarcastic about clichés or outdated expressions, but he just said, "sure."

"Well, let's go then. This setup offers two different kinds of virtual reality training. The first is all done in the computer. The computer will put an image on the screen. You take your instruments, put them through the permanent 'incisions' in your virtual patient, and operate. The computer will sense the movements of the instruments and respond by showing you a digital image of what would have happened if it was real tissue in a real patient."

"Let me show you an example. Look at the monitor." John pushed a few keys and the image of an actual pelvis came up. It had probably come from a tape of an actual operation. Some endoscopic surgeons tape every operation. The tapes can be used for teaching, for reference or they can be sent to the referring doctor. Some patients even like to have a copy for themselves.

Dackel didn't tape anything. He did very few endoscopic procedures, mostly laparoscopy for tying tubes or trying to figure out why someone was in pain. If he found a problem, he would generally remove the scope and make a traditional incision.

"Okay Dr. Dackel, here's your first task. Tie her tubes."

Dackel breathed a mental sigh of relief. This he knew how to do. He took a telescope from the table, inserted it through a ready made incision in the dummy's navel and into a hollow body cavity. But as soon as the scope went in, the picture began to move as if he were actually looking around in this patient's pelvis. He moved the scope to the left, and the left ovary and tube came into view. He moved it to the right and there was the right side. He moved it up a little higher and saw the appendix.

"This is remarkable!" he said. "How do you do this?"

"The technology is pretty simple to explain, Dr. Dackel. We gathered images from thousands of videotaped operations and from the Visible Human Project, and digitally fed them into a computer, which can call up any one of them in a fraction of a second. The instruments you are working with are all wired into the same computer. There are also sensors in the mannequin that help the computer figure out where your instruments are. When you move the telescope, for example, the computer brings up the image of whatever you would be looking at in this pelvis. When you grasp the tube with the forceps, which you will do next, the computer will figure that out and switch to a picture of a tube being grasped. Actually, your instrument won't be grasping anything. There are no organs in the mannequin."

"Remarkable, let me try," said Dackel.

He looked at the instruments on the table and chose a Kleppinger bipolar forceps, the instrument he usually used for tubal sterilization. Tying tubes is an old expression. Many people think that the fallopian tube is actually tied in a knot. Actually, most tubal sterilizations these days are done by one of two methods. They are fulgurated or burned with electrical energy, or they are occluded with an elastic band or a metal clip. Tying is sometimes involved, if the abdomen is opened for another reason, like a Caesarian or an ovarian cyst, but even then it is a suture that is tied around the tube.

Dackel expertly guided the Kleppingers to the left tube, picked it up in its mid-portion and pressed a pedal on the floor. He heard the familiar tone indicating that the current was on. He watched as the tissue in the jaws of his instrument turned white, a sign that the tube was being rendered functionless.

"Absolutely amazing," he said, over and over.

"You did that very well," said John.

That made Dackel feel good. Somehow the fact that he was being praised by a 37-year-old salesman who had probably never even seen a live operation didn't really matter. Dackel was not very confident about his endoscopic skills but the truth was he was probably better at it than he thought. Laparoscopy had just started to become popular in the United States at about the time he finished his residency, so instead of learning it over his three year training program like he learned all his other surgical skills, his introduction to the technique was a two day workshop similar to this one.

"Are you ready to try some endoscopic knot tying?"

"Not really," said Dackel, his balloon of accomplishment starting to deflate. I've never done it before."

Duke seemed puzzled. He had been told by the educational coordinator that Dackel was well trained in endoscopic surgery, as was everyone attending the course.

"Would you like me to show you how?"

"Okay," said Dackel, "I guess it couldn't hurt."

John picked up a laparoscopic needle driver and a needle that had a wire attached to it instead of suture. He inserted it through a port on the lower abdomen just above and to the right of the amazingly realistic but nonetheless fake pubic hairline. He put a grasper through a similar incision on the left. The screen showed the two instruments with a normal purple suture in place of the wire. John deftly turned his wrist and the monitor showed the suture going through the top of the uterus. As expected, tiny rivulets of blood started streaming from both the entrance and the exit needle holes. Duke grasped the needle with the grasper on the left, wrapped the "suture" around the needle driver three times and then grasped the tail of the suture with the needle holder. When he pulled the instruments apart, Dackel saw the virtual knot tighten and the bleeding stop.

"It's so hard to grasp the fact that we're looking at a video tape and the instruments we're seeing aren't the ones we're using," said Dackel.

"It's not really a tape," said John. "It may have come from a tape, but the computer has digitized it into millions of images."

"Whatever," said Dackel. "Let me try."

Duke hit a few keys and a fresh pelvis appeared on the screen. Dackel picked up the needle driver and the wired needle. He made several attempts to drive the needle into his target, but he didn't seem to have the eye-hand coordination that it took. Duke took Al's hands and guided them until it finally worked. Dackel just looked at him.

"What do I do now?" he asked helplessly.

Duke, sensing the frustration of his student, said, "You know, you really don't need to know how to tie sutures to use the DAC-III. Why don't we just kill a few more tubes."

Duke was a good salesman. After a few more attempts, John said, "Let's try some hysteroscopy."

"John, let me tell you something you may not know about me." said Dackel sheepishly, "I don't have a lot of experience with hysteroscopy."

Somehow Duke wasn't surprised, but he was somewhat upset. The company was about to launch the biggest breakthrough in gynecologic surgery in years. They met for months in strategy sessions and decided that they wanted to introduce the DAC-III through the leaders in the gynecologic community. They had already invested 40 million in the training facility and were ready to spend another 40 in advertising, training and demonstration equipment. Dackel was probably a decent surgeon, but he was the furthest thing from what the company had envisioned as a DAC-III pioneer.

"Have you read the monograph on hysteroscopy that was in your packet?"

"I didn't see one, they must have left it out," he lied.

Duke knew he was lying.

"Well then let's start at the beginning. "

Duke went to the bottom of the table and positioned the mannequin's legs in the stirrups. Dackel couldn't get over how real her vulva looked. He prayed that he wouldn't twitch. He didn't.

"You start by putting the speculum into the vagina the usual way. Will you do that for me Dr.?"

"Sure," Dackel said as he expertly placed the instrument the way he had done it hundreds of thousands of time in the past.

"Now grasp the cervix with a tenaculum."

Dackel picked up a long instrument that can best be compared to a pair of miniature ice tongs, not the kind at the dinner table, but rather the ones that the ice men used to carry the big blocks of ice. He clamped it onto the top rim of the cervix.

"Before you put the scope in, Dr. Dackel, it's important to run the DAC-III through the self diagnostic cycle and test fire it. These two buttons must be pushed simultaneously to test fire the DAC-III. Why don't you go ahead and aim the wand at the test target and push the both of them at once."

Dackel held the wand carefully a few inches above a container of synthetic tissue that looked like Jell-O and pushed the button labeled "Test." Nothing happened.

"Doc, remember, you have to push both buttons at the same time in order to test fire. It's kind of like on a tape recorder, you have to push record and play at the same time. It's a safety feature. I'll tell you what, you aim the scope at the test target, and I'll push the buttons."

Dackel aimed the wand once again. Before Duke hit the buttons he explained what was going to happen.

"This test firing is just for the treatment cycle. The mapping function doesn't need to be tested. First the MR will line up the protons in the atoms, then the ultrasound waves will be generated, and finally the laser will be fired. Only when they hit the target at the same time will you see an effect. The other thing is that the power density during the test fire is pretty high. You never want to test fire when you are in the uterus because you can do some real damage, so be careful. And always wear your safety goggles because if you forget where you're aiming this thing, it will take out your eye pretty easily."

Dackel held the scope steady and Duke pushed the buttons. There was a whirring noise that lasted just a second or so, and then a flash of light. The power sources combined to blast a perfectly round 5 millimeter wide crater that was exactly 4 millimeters deep. There was no charring, and just a wisp of smoke. Dackel was impressed.

"The next step would normally be to dilate the cervix up to 9 millimeters, but the one on the dummy is already dilated. Now turn on the fluid flow and insert the hysteroscope. Watch the screen, Doctor, watch the screen while you're putting it in so you'll know where you are. You'll see how the fluid will distend the uterus like a balloon as it flows through the scope."

Dackel turned his head toward the monitor. He was familiar with the technique of inserting things into the uterus. D&C's and abortions both required that instruments be inserted, but he had always done it blindly, by feel. This was the first time he was able to actually able to see where he was going. He watched as the scope went through the narrow cervix. It looked like a tunnel. Suddenly, on the screen, an image of the inside of the uterus appeared.

"Wow, it looks just like in the books," Dackel said almost gleefully. This wasn't so hard. Look at the lining. You can actually see the endometrium and look, there's the opening to the left tube."

"You're doing great, Dr. Dackel," said Duke. "You're a natural."

What he had done to this point was not really difficult for someone with his surgical experience. The difficult part comes when actual surgery needs to be performed in the uterus. The DAC-III, if it worked like they promised, would allow a surgeon with just basic abilities to do what formerly required great skill and practice. In a sense, Dackel was the doctor for whom the DAC-III was designed.

"Now suppose this patient was a bleeder and you couldn't control her with hormones, and you've done a D&C and the tissue was benign. What would you do?"

"Well, up 'till today, I would have done a hysterectomy, but I suspect you're going to change my mind, right?" said Dackel, feeling confident that he was about to learn an *alterrrnative*.

"I'm certainly going to try," said Duke. "I'm going to activate the DAC-III. It will take a few seconds. It's very important that you keep the scope still. This gizmo anchors it to the tenaculum so it doesn't move during the scanning. Ready? Watch the screen."

Dackel watched as green lines rapidly criss-crossed the picture on the monitor, first vertically, then horizontally, then diagonally in both directions. There were so many lines that eventually he couldn't see the tissue.

"This is why it's important to keep the scope still," said Duke. "It has nothing to do with the scan, the computer can correct for that. It's because you lose your view for a few seconds and if you move the scope, you might perforate."

Dackel knew all about perforations. A perforation occurs when an instrument tears or pierces through the muscular wall of the uterus. "Perforation is a known and accepted complication of any intrauterine surgery," he would tell his patients when he was giving them his informed consent lecture.

He thought about the first time it happened to him. He was an intern assisting on a D&C. Actually, he wasn't assisting at all. You don't need an assistant on a D&C. It is basically a one person procedure. Medical training is often "see one, do one, teach one." That case was his first "do one."

He passed one of the dilators, the metal instrument that stretches the cervix open to allow the curette or scraping instrument in, and the dilator just kept going. His teacher took over, and, as with most perfs, everything turned out all right. There was no excessive bleeding and very little chance of injury to the intestines because the perforation had been done with a blunt instrument.

After the case, and Dackel's attack of diarrhea, a reaction that he still experienced when faced with a surgical complication, his professor called him in to his office to calm him down.

"Al, the only way anyone can learn how hard to push is to push too hard once or twice. You know, there are three kinds of gynecologists, the kind that's perforated a uterus, the kind that hasn't perforated yet and the kind that lies about it."

Dackel cut short his reminiscence when he saw the lines on the monitor disappear and the picture of the inside of the uterus return. He had trouble remembering that this was a virtual recreation of the operation and that his scope was inside a hollow plastic doll.

"Watch this," said Duke as he pushed the "display model" button on the DAC-III control panel. The screen then changed to a color map of the uterus. It looked three dimensional, as if you could almost see through the tissues.

"This is the inner surface view. What you're seeing is the endometrium. Notice that if you place the cursor on the endometrium, the word 'endometrium' appears in the upper left hand corner of the screen, and just in case you want to use a tape of a procedure for teaching or education, in parenthesis, next to 'endometrium' it says 'inner lining of the uterus.' Would you like to see the muscular layer underneath?"

Dackel sat there staring at the screen with his mouth open. He shook his head affirmatively.

Duke pushed a button and the screen changed, highlighting the muscle layer as clearly as a Netter drawing. Another button, and the blood vessels were highlighted.

"Now, suppose we want to stop this woman's bleeding forever," said Duke switching back to the endometrial view. "All we have to do is tell the DAC-III to go to work."

He returned to the picture highlighting the endometrium, simultaneously pushed the two "TREAT" buttons and within a few minutes the endometrium turned from a healthy pink to a dull beige and the screen flashed the message, "TREATMENT COMPLETED."

"It's as simple as that, Dr. Dackel, but before we get out of here, I want to go over some very important safety issues. First of all, although the laser is contained in the unit and the fiberoptic cables are all safety coated, we suggest laser safety goggles for everyone in the operating room and eye patches for the patient, just in case. As far as the magnet emulator in the MRI, you don't have to worry about ferrous metals like with the old fashioned MRI machines, but you do have to be careful with any machinery that may be magnet sensitive. Your anesthesiologist will need to be aware of the fact that you're using the device."

"The other things that you need to worry about are just the usual hysteroscopy precautions. We discussed perforation. The other one is water intoxication. They're going to cover that tomorrow in the troubleshooting and safety lecture. Well, we're through here. Do you have any questions?"

Dackel was overwhelmed. He was excited at the prospect of, for the first time in 25 years, being on the cutting edge of anything. He was optimistic that this could save his practice and, that when those bastards at QHM find out that he has the only machine in town, they'll come crawling to him. But he was also scared. He had done his first hysteroscopy today and it was on a plastic doll. The virtual reality training was impressive, but would it be different with a real patient? He was tired. He needed a nap.

Chapter 10

Like a child after a hard day at the zoo, Alfred Dackel, with his eyes heavy and his mind almost off, walked in slow motion back to the van. He fell asleep during the short ride back to the hotel, and the driver had to wake him when they got there. Dackel went up to his room, stripped to his jockey shorts and crashed on the bed. He awoke at 8:30 that evening to some laughing in the hall. He was starved. He took a peach and a nectarine from the basket of fruit and when he finished them he went back for the banana. He tried to call Carrie again but there was no answer. Then he called Arlene.

"Hillowww," she answered in the pseudo sophisticated voice she used when she was trying very hard to deny her South Philadelphia roots.

"Hi, what's going on?" he said, as tenderly as anything he ever said to her.

"Oh, Al, you wouldn't believe what's going on around here." He could tell by her tone and the length of the breath she took that she was warming up for a big one. Dackel could tell when she was about to begin one of her famous epic narratives because she always warmed up her voice, almost like a pitcher winds up before he unleashes his best fast ball.

"First of all, Al, you know Sara across the street? Well, her gardener was in an accident so he called and said that there was no way he could do her lawn today, and you know they're having that party tonight, which, by the way Al, I am not happy about going to alone. Well, anyway, I said why don't you call that other gardener, you know, the one that..."

Dackel let her go on. He figured that she probably waited all day to tell him about this major turbulence that will, no doubt, become an important chapter in Hanford Lane history. He let her go on but he didn't really listen. He thought instead about Angel or Carrie or whatever her name was. She was really a nice girl and she seemed bright too. It must be nice to have those attributes and also be able to turn men on to the point that they give you money just to be teased.

"...So, P.S., both gardeners get there at the same time and they get into this terrible fist fight..."

What if Carrie was pregnant? He really couldn't help her. There was a combination of medications that can cause an abortion, but the patient needs to be carefully monitored for several days. Besides he didn't have a Florida license. Then he started thinking about the way she was shaved. Why did that turn him on so much? Because it was different? Because it reminded him of a child? He hoped not. It certainly didn't do anything for him in the office. Red was preoccupied with pubic hair design. He was constantly asking Dackel about patients that he knew and what kind of pubic hair they had. His philosophy was that women who "groomed" down there thought about sex more than women who didn't. He further assumed that they were hotter and therefore more promiscuous. He had no personal experience on which to base this theory, but nonetheless, he was confident that the committee would someday recognize its brilliance and award him the first Nobel *Piece* Prize.

Dackel himself was intrigued with the variety of styles and cuts he had observed over the years. He had learned that some of them had names. The "landing strip" was one of his favorites. This was a thin strip of midline hair, not exceeding an inch in width. There was also the "treasure trail." This was usually present in a hairy unshaved woman. Basically it was a strip of hair starting at the belly button and trailing down the lower abdomen to the "treasure."

He even made up some names of his own. Three of them honored his all time favorite cinema heroes. The "Curly" was, of course, a totally shaved vulva, the "Larry" was just the opposite, and the "Moe" was a name he reserved for many Asians and anyone else with straight pubic hair.

He agreed with Klee, to some extent, with regard to the personality of "Curly" women, but he also knew that some women shaved themselves to get rid of crabs.

"...so then the policeman said to her, 'Look lady, which one of these guys do you want to cut the lawn,' so she started crying..."

He said "um hm" a few times and finally cut her off. He had to. There was no estimating how long she could go on uninterrupted. No one had ever let her.

"Listen, Arlene, I gotta go. Do me a favor and call Gene Porter at home. Just make sure everything's okay with my practice. If he needs me, tell him to call me at the hotel. I left the number on my desk in the den. I'm gonna go to dinner now and then maybe get together with some of the other doctors. I'll call you tomorrow." He quickly hung up.

Dackel knew that he couldn't give her an opportunity to respond to anything if he ever wanted to get off the phone. Had he done so, he was sure he would have heard about Sherry Porter's face lift, he would have been lectured about what he should and shouldn't eat for dinner, and he would have been asked to describe the other conference participants, especially what they were wearing compared to his outfits. He hated it when she referred to his clothes as "outfits."

He showered, put on the same white pants and the same shirt he had worn the night before, and went down to the hotel restaurant. Most of the other people from the conference had gotten together in groups for dinner. Some stayed at the hotel, and others ventured out to check out the Tampa night life.

He ate a barbecue sampler platter consisting of a rack of baby backs, a chicken breast (white meat is low in fat, he rationalized) and barbecued shrimp. He had his choice of baked potato or French fries and, of course, he went with the fries. Because he missed out on the creme brulee for lunch, he wanted one for dinner, but this restaurant didn't offer it so he settled for chocolate chip amoretto cheesecake and a cup of cappuccino. On his way out he took a handful and a half of mints and put the handful in his pocket and the half in his mouth.

He went out to the car and took off for Scampers. It was a lot more crowded than it was the previous night and there seemed to be more dancers. He paid his cover and asked the bouncer nearest the door if Angel had been on yet. He learned that she would be there in about an hour. Dackel felt some excitement but he was majorly confused about what to do about it. He was sure that he wanted to see her again, but he was really not sure where he wanted it to go from there. All he knew was that he liked how she made him feel. But what was he going to do about it?

Oh God, he said to himself, I'm thinking like Arlene talks. Then he thought about Arlene, and he felt guilty for even questioning what he would do. I'm married, he said to himself, and that's that.

He looked at his watch. She would be on in 55 minutes. The dancer on stage was heavier than most he had seen, in fact she was downright fat. Nonetheless, she went through all the mandatory maneuvers: lying on back with feet spread up in air; bending over and looking at customer through legs; walking on elbows and knees; and rubbing crotch on pole (brass pole on stage, not ethnic customer). She was actually pretty good, good enough, in fact, to earn a dollar from Dackel. He went up to the stage to put it between naked breasts but when he got close, he could see that she was all sweaty. He attempted to make his deposit without getting his hand trapped, but he lost. When she finally let him go, his hand was soaked. He was grossed out. He wiped it on the front of his pants and then realized that she must have been wearing body make-up, because his hand left a large, flesh toned blotch on the front of whiter than white pants.

He went into the men's room to try to get the stain out, but all he managed to do was to spread it around and soak his pants in the process. He looked around for one of those hand blowers but all they had were paper towels. His choices were to wait it out in the well lighted john until his pants dried or go back to his table where it was dark. He thought he would be less obvious at his table.

What he didn't count on was the dancer who had just started. She liked to dance in black light, the kind of light that makes white stand out like neon. Under these lighting conditions, Dackel's pants lit up. The stain stood out even more and the wet part looked soaked.

"Dr. Dackel," he heard from a table right outside the men's room, "glad you could join us."

The voice came from a group of about twelve. Five National salesmen, and seven doctors, one of whom was Dr. Mary McLeod. Dackel panicked. He thought about going back into the bathroom but he realized that it would just make it worse, so he just stood there for a moment totally frazzled and with as much control as a deer in the quality control lab of a headlight factory. What could he say? How foolish did he look?

"Spill some coffee on your pants?" asked Bill Horn. Boy, was he good. He knew it didn't look anything like a coffee stain, and he knew that everyone else knew that it didn't look anything like a coffee stain, but he figured that asking that question would allow all of them to get out of what he realized was a "sticky situation." It would have worked too if Dr. Mary hadn't started drinking at the hotel three hours earlier.

"Coffee, my ass, it looks to me like he's just having a good time," she said, barely getting the words out through the coughter (a combination of coughing and laughter.)

No one said anything. Even Horn, the salesman's salesman couldn't think of a way out of this one. Everyone except McLeod was embarrassed. Dackel was mortified.

"It is coffee," he blustered, as he walked out of the club. Horn took off after him.

Dr. Mary McLeod was an excellent doctor. She had pioneered many hysteroscopic and laparoscopic procedures and had invented several instruments that bore her name: the McLeod Myoma Debulker; the McLeod Cyst Extractor and the McLeod Polyp Snare to name a few. She was also a prolific author, an in-demand lecturer and a popular teacher. She did almost everything well except hold her liquor. She didn't drink often because she knew what it did to her. Alcohol gave her inhibitions the night off.

"What did I say?" she yelled rhetorically. "What's up with him? This is a strip club, not a fucking church. So what if he came in his goddamn pants, that's not against the law. C'mon let's enjoy ourselves."

Mary was the only female patron in the club. She had never been to a nudie bar before and if she hadn't gotten shit-faced at dinner, she probably wouldn't have been in this one. But she was here and she was going to have fun.

"Give me a vodka martini with an onion," she yelled to the cocktail waitress. "On second thought, make that two onions. I'm not going to kiss anyone tonight."

Dr. Haddad was hoping she was wrong.

Bill Horn caught up with Dackel in the parking lot. He tried to convince him to come back into the club.

"She's drunk, Dr. Dackel. She looks like the foolish one, not you. She was just making a joke at your expense. Everyone wants you to come on back in."

Dackel thanked him for his words and then got into his car and went back to the hotel. His message light was on. He dialed the operator and waited at least a million rings before a perky voice full of sunshine answered, "front desk."

"Messages for Dr. Dackel," he growled.

"Yes doctor, you have two. At 9:30 your wife called. The message is that there is a squirrel in the house and she doesn't know what to do or who to call. Also at 9:50 you got a call from a Carrie. She didn't leave her last name. She said she will be dancing at Scampers tonight and she hopes you can come."

"Thanks," he barely said before hanging up. Then he said to himself, almost out loud, "She *hopes* I can come, and the rest of the world thinks I already *did*."

He was certainly not in the mood to listen to Arlene telling him in eleven different ways that there was a squirrel in the house, so he decided not to call her back. He called Carrie's apartment in case there was the remote chance that she had gotten an answering machine in the past few hours. She hadn't. He tried calling Scampers but they wouldn't put him through to her, so he just went to sleep.

At 3 AM his phone rang. He was disoriented and thought for a second that he was at home and it was a patient. He was used to getting calls in the middle of the night and he realized early on that very few of them were emergencies. Women would call with urinary burning or vaginal itching knowing full well that even if he could diagnose them over the telephone, the drug store wouldn't open until 8 o'clock.

"Dr. Dackel," he said into the wrong end of the receiver. "Hello, hello." He finally figured out what was going on and where he was. He turned the receiver. "Dr. Dackel."

"Dr. Dackel, it's Carrie. I'm sorry to wake you but I didn't see you at the club today and I'm having a problem and you're the only one I can talk to." She had tears in her voice. "Please, will you help me?"

"What kind of trouble, Carrie?" Dackel asked, concerned about her problem, but at the same time aware that he was becoming much more involved with this situation than he should be.

"My boyfriend came back tonight when I was at the club. He saw the pregnancy test in my bathroom and he went nuts. He wants to get married and have the baby."

"The test was positive?" asked Dackel.

"I don't know, I didn't even take it yet."

"Well then what are you upset about."

"I told him that I didn't want to marry him and if I was pregnant, I was going to have an abortion. He beat me up Dr. Dackel. He hit me." Her last word morphed into a hysterical cry, the kind that comes not just from the eyes, but from the whole body. It was the kind of deep exhausting cry that physical pain can't even cause. This cry could come only from a direct hit to the center of the soul. He heard Arlene cry like that only once, when her best friend died of ovarian cancer.

"Where is he now?" Dackel asked when she regained a few degrees of composure.

"He left a few minutes ago."

"Did you call the police?"

"No, I just called you-u-u-u." the words turning into convulsive sobbing.

"Carrie, tell me where you live, I'll come right over."

She gave him the address of her apartment and the code to get into the gate.

"Call the police, Carrie, I'll be right over."

He got dressed, brushed his teeth and was in the car in less than five minutes. He got directions from the night bellman and was at her apartment in 15 minutes.

Her apartment was clean and furnished tastefully, but not expensively. He didn't pay much attention when he came in, but he did see shelves of books, CDs and videotapes. She had a top of the line Sony Trinitron TV and what looked like two Sony VCR's stacked one on the other.

"Are you okay? Did you call the police?"

Her eyes were a little red but she wasn't crying any more. She was wearing a fluffy white terrycloth robe, like the kind they supply in hotel suites. He guessed that that's where hers came from.

"I didn't call. I'm going to wait till tomorrow and call my lawyer. I'm just so scared."

"Do you think he'll come back tonight?" asked Dackel, as afraid for himself as he was for her.

"I know he won't," she answered. "He's a truck driver and I know he has to be in Miami by the morning. Dr. Dackel, will you stay with me tonight? Please."

"Carrie, I really can't. I came over to see if you were hurt, and it looks like you're okay. I'd like to help more, but I really can't. Why don't we call the police."

"It wouldn't do any good," she said with tears starting to well up. "His brother's a cop. I've called before and they never do anything."

"Honey, you don't look like you need a doctor tonight. Maybe you could call a girlfriend."

"Dr. Dackel, please just look where he hit me and make sure I'm all right."

"Sure," said Dackel, who couldn't believe that he was in an apartment with a stripper who just invited him to spend the night, "let's have a look."

Carrie untied the sash and instead of discretely exposing the injured part of her body, she let the whole robe slip off of her shoulders and onto the floor.

God, she's sexy even under these circumstances, he thought to himself, finding it somewhat strange that she did what she did, but realizing that she was used to being naked.

"He hit me right here," she said pointing to her left breast, "and I think I feel a lump."

"I don't see a bruise," said Dackel, "but it may not show up until tomorrow. The lump may be a hematoma. Let me see."

He bent over to look more closely at the breast and touched it gently and professionally.

"I don't feel anything," he said, and then he cupped the breast with his other hand to give it support so he could examine it better. "No, Carrie, I think you're okay." He picked up her robe and handed it to her just as he would have done in his office after he finished an examination. He even turned his back to give her the opportunity to put it on, but she didn't.

"He also kicked me here," she said pointing to her pelvis.

"Carrie, I'm a little uncomfortable for some reason. I mean I do this every day, but the circumstances..."

"Dr. Dackel, please just check, I'll even pay you."

"That won't be necessary. Okay, lie down and I'll see what I can see.

She walked over to the sofa and slowly sat down as if she were favoring her back. She swung her feet up and propped her head with a pillow.

"Where did he kick you?" he asked.

She made circular movements around the area of where her pubic hair would have been if she had any.

"Does it hurt? he asked.

"Yes, right here," she said continuing the circles.

He sat on the edge of the sofa and carefully palpated her lower abdomen and mons pubis, pressing gently and then more firmly, all the time watching her face for cues that would give him an idea where the pain was located and how severe it was. He was careful not to touch her clitoral area. If it hurt, he felt, she would direct him there.

"I think you're going to be fine." he said, "I don't think he did any damage. Put some ice on the tender areas tonight. You might feel sore tomorrow, and if things seem like they're getting worse, see your doctor on Monday."

"Dr. Dackel, I can't thank you enough. Could I ask one more favor? I know it's late."

"I really have to get going..."

"This is really easy, will you do the pregnancy test for me?"

"Okay, give me a urine specimen."

She went into the bathroom, still without the robe. She didn't shut the door.

"Doctor Dackel, I'm so dumb, I forgot the paper cup. Could you get one for me. They're in the top cabinet in the kitchen, the one all the way to the left."

He went into the kitchen and found the cups. He tried to hand her one at arm's length, attempting to stay out of the bathroom, but she didn't get up to meet him halfway, so he stepped in and gave it to her. She dropped it and it rolled away so he picked it up and handed it to her once again. Dackel was actually becoming more comfortable being alone with a naked stripper, but watching her try to pee in a cup was a little too much for him. He closed the door and waited until he heard a flush.

"Where is the test?" he asked.

"It's in here," she said walking towards the bedroom.

He followed her in and she handed him the test.

"It's really quite simple," he explained. "You just take the dropper and put a few drops of urine in this chamber right here." In less than a minute a single blue line became visible indicating that she was not pregnant. If she had been, a plus sign would have appeared.

"You're okay, he said coming over and sitting on the side of the bed next to where she had laid down, "See this negative sign?"

"Where?" she said, pulling herself up by putting an arm on his shoulder. "Oh, I see."

"I've got to leave now," said Dackel, "You'll be okay."

"You're not leaving without a hug." she said, "You're the best doctor."

She hugged him and he hugged her back, and despite the fact she was naked, he didn't even get a twitch. He let himself out and drove back to the hotel. It was close to 5:30 A.M. when he got back into bed.

Chapter 11

He must have slept through the alarm, or maybe he didn't set it right, or at all, but it wasn't until after ten that he woke up.

Shit, I finally come to a course that has something to teach me and I miss half of it, he thought while he brushed his teeth.

He dressed quickly, without showering or shaving, and drove over to the lab. He got there at 10:30. He had been assigned to group B and was supposed to have been in the lab for the first part of the morning. The agenda was to go through some basic hysteroscopic procedures, and learn more about the equipment, how to set it up and how to troubleshoot it. It is essential that a surgeon knows how to set up, break down and adjust any instrument he works with. Most of the time the nurses can do it better, but occasionally you get a new nurse or the one that's working with you isn't familiar with the tools.

He got there in time for the coffee break.

"Dr. Dackel, I'm terribly sorry about last night," said Bill Horn. "I hope that's not what kept you away this morning."

Dackel had actually forgotten about the events of the early evening.

"Nah, I make it a policy never to let a drunk upset me," he said, loud enough for Mary McLeod to hear him.

"Touché," she replied, shrugging her shoulders and raising her eyebrows with a "shit happens" expression.

He glanced her way and mentally gave her the finger.

"I overslept," he said, "pure and simple. I really am sorry I missed the session."

"That's okay Dr. Dackel, you must have good connections because the boss is arranging a private tutoring session in your own operating room once the equipment arrives. He also decided to invite you to be one of our clinical investigators and that means you can have the machine for at least a year at no cost to you or your hospital. He recognizes talent when he sees it."

Those were Horn's words. His thoughts were a little different. He couldn't imagine why the brass would want to waste a million-dollar machine on someone who's not only an amateur, but an asshole. Dackel had pretty much the same thoughts.

He ate his breakfast while everyone else had a coffee break. Dave Evans announced that group B was to follow him to the studio.

They got on an elevator and went down to the basement to a room marked "Studio One." It was a large room with television cameras and wires all over the floor and lights hanging from everywhere on the ceiling. He felt intimidated just as Evans had predicted in his lecture.

"Let me introduce you to your floor manager, Steve Sachs," said Evans. "He's going to give you a quick orientation before we start."

Start what, thought Dackel. What are we starting?

"Hi," said Steve, "This is the studio, but I guess you figured that out by now [polite laughter]. Over there, that platform with the desk and chairs is the first set. That's where you'll do the first scene of the video. You can see, behind the set, is a painting we call a flat. We have several that we can move in to make it seem more like your office. If your office is in the city, we have a city scene. If you're out in the country, we have one of those too. We have a high-rise flat and one that looks like you're on ground level. It won't be exact, of course, but for this scene, most of what we'll need will be tight shots of you."

What scene? Why am I the only one who doesn't know what the hell he's talking about? Thought Dackel to himself. Why don't I ever know what's going on?

"For the second scene we'll go to this set which hopefully looks enough like an operating room to fool your patients. We'll dress you up in a gown and mask and you'll pretend you're doing a hysteroscopy on this dummy. I know she looks like plastic now, but she'll look real on the tape. So let's get started. It should only take a few minutes for each scene."

He divided the group into two and led each half to their set. Dackel went to the O.R. set first and before he knew it, he was in a gown, gloves, hat and mask.

"All you have to do is sit here Doctor, and look through the hysteroscope," said a production assistant who introduced herself as Allison. "We won't be recording any sound so I'll just tell you what to do."

Dackel sat down on the stool and for the second time in his life, held a hysteroscope in his hand.

"Now move it from side to side a little like you're inspecting the endometrial cavity - and in and out. Not quite that much doctor."

Christ, she knows more than me, he thought.

"That's better - now once more. That's good. And we're done. Who's next?"

He watched as the others took their turns. He got a kick out of watching Haddad who kept looking at the camera and smiling through his mask despite Allison's direction.

After twenty minutes or so, the group was finished. They walked over to the other set to see what they would be doing next. Dackel still wasn't sure what was going on, so he went over to Allison and quietly asked her to fill him in.

"What we're going to do is make an educational and informed consent video tape. Most of it has been professionally done, but you will introduce the tape and then, when we show the operation, it will look like you're doing it.

"Isn't that dishonest?" he asked.

"No, you will be the one doing your patient's surgery and we can't come into everyone's O.R. to get you on tape. Besides, it will be comforting to the patient to see you with the instrument, and if you want, you can tell her that this was only a simulation."

He felt better, but then he realized he hadn't shaved and he was wearing one of his stretched out Izods. He went back to Allison.

"Listen, I got up kind of late today and I didn't get a chance to shave or anything, and this shirt..."

"Don't worry Doctor, we have a shirt and a lab coat for you. Justine will take care of you. You'll look fine."

At the moment, Justine was struggling with Mary McLeod's hair. It looked like the hair was winning.

"Watch the others Doctor, it's really easy," said Allison.

Dackel walked up behind one of the big cameras and watched someone he hadn't met looking straight at the camera and talking about ablation.

"He went over to Allison again.

"How will I know what to say?" he asked her with a little panic in his voice.

"It's all on the TelePrompTer," she giggled. "All you have to do is read."

"TelePrompTer?" he said, "I don't know how to work a TelePrompTer."

"There's nothing to know, all you do is read. We'll follow at your pace. Besides, it's only a few sentences. I promise, you'll do fine."

He watched a few more doctors take their turns until Justine came and got him. She spent a few minutes looking him over before she said anything.

"Doctor, are you starting a beard or are you trying for the Don Johnson look?" she asked.

"Who's Don Johnson?" he snapped back.

"Oh, I'm sorry," she said laughing. "He's an actor. He played a cop on Miami Vice a few years ago, and he always had a five o'clock shadow. The look became very popular for a while. I wouldn't suggest it for you, but you would look great in a full beard."

"If God wanted men to have beards, he wouldn't have invented razors!" Dackel snapped. He was serious.

"Do you use a blade or an electric?"

"Never used an electric in my life."

"Come into the dressing room, I have a disposable BiC for you. You'll have to use soap though because I don't have any shaving cream."

"I've done it before."

"And while you're back there, take off your shirt. I'll give you one from wardrobe."

"Can I ask a stupid question?" said Dackel, "How is it that you happen to have extra shirts around?"

"For situations just like this one, Doctor. National covers all the bases."

"They sure do," he thought as he went into the dressing room. He took off his shirt and shaved with what little lather he could work up from the hand soap. He was done and his shirt had not yet arrived. Bare chested, he went to look for Justine. She was on her way to the dressing room with a garment bag.

"Here are a few different sizes," she said, looking at his big fat hairy belly and trying to not look as repulsed as she was. See if you can find one that will fit."

"Thanks, just hold onto it for a second while I unzip this thing," Dackel said, struggling with the zipper on the garment bag. "There. This one looks about right."

He put it on and went over to watch some more of the taping.

Just before it was his turn, Justine gave him a paisley tie and a white coat. She took a triangular shaped white sponge and covered his face with pancake makeup. There was nothing that she could do about his hair, but she powdered his head so it wouldn't shine.

"I feel like a woman," he said, "when are you going to give me some breasts?"

Justine laughed. "Don't worry, this is the same makeup I use on Clint Eastwood."

It was time for Dackel to make his movie debut. He took his seat.

Evans was directing this scene.

"Okay, Dr. DackEL, I mean Dr. DACkel. Gee, that's the second time I did that. I do apologize. Dr. Dackel, the words are on this screen right here on the front of this camera. Try to keep you head still and just read them as if you were having a conversation with a patient. Very relaxed, almost casual. You can start any time you're ready."

"Ahmmm," Dackel cleared his throat, "Hello, I'm..."

"Hold it, Doctor, it's okay to clear your throat before you begin but if you do, wait a few seconds before you start to talk. That way we'll be able to cut it out."

"I'm sorry."

"No, it's quite all right, just begin again."

"Ready?"

"Any time doctor."

"Hello I'm state name...Oh for Christ's sake, I'm sorry. I can't believe I did that. I'll start again. Hello, I'm Dr. Alfred Dackel..."

"Hold on," Dr. Dackel, "You seem to be squinting, do you wear glasses?"

"Sometimes I do, but I lost them last night. They were expensive too, I think I paid three hundred bucks for them."

"That's no problem." He pressed a button on a box that he had clipped to his waist. "Donny, can you up the font size on the prompter? Thanks."

The words suddenly doubled in size. Now there were only a few on a line, but he was easily able to see them.

"Can you see the words now Doctor?"

"Wow, they're nice and big, I don't think I'll have a problem."

"Okay, then, here we go. Any time you're ready Doctor."

"Hello, I'm Dr. Alfred Dackel, and I want you to meet a good friend of mine, Dr. Mark MacDonald, the Medical Director of National Medical Innovations, the company that developed and manufactures the DAC-III. Dr. MacDonald will explain how this unique and wonderful instrument will help me when I perform your endometrial ablation surgery."

"That was good Dr. Dackel. Now let's do it again, and this time lean forward in you chair a little, and don't interlace your fingers, just rest one hand on top of the other. And doctor, try not to lick your lips once you start. Do you need a glass of water?"

"Maybe, I'm a little dry."

Someone brought him a glass of water. He took a sip and then promptly spilled the rest on his lap.

"It looks like I wet my pants," Dackel laughed.

"Don't worry, Doctor, we're shooting you from the chest up."

"De ja vu all over again," said Mary McLeod.

Dackel read the lines a few more times and didn't do a bad job. He went back to the dressing room and took off the shirt. Justine walked into the room surprising him because she didn't knock. Luckily all she caught him doing was scrubbing his face with wet paper towels.

"You'll be scrubbing all day with those," she said. "Try this." She handed him some Albolene. "It will work much better."

He dipped his finger into the jar and scooped out a glob, which he rubbed all over his face.

"Now I really feel like a girl with all this grease. Why don't just you give me a pair of panties."

"Dr. Dackel, you're too funny," she said, trying very hard to hide her sarcasm, but probably not succeeding.

When everyone was finished taping, the group went back up to the main conference room. Jerry Edmonds was at the podium.

"Well I hope you ladies and gentlemen enjoyed this weekend and I also hope that now you are all as excited as we are about the DAC-III. Doctors, you have been hand picked from around the country to be the first to try the DAC-III system. As we've said, we're starting slowly, but within the year we hope to have approval for DAC-III treatment of fibroids and within three years, doctors, we, or should I say you, will be treating most cancers of the female reproductive tract with the DAC-III Sonomagnetic Laser. I sincerely hope that you will stay with us for the ride. Our commitment to you is that we will always be there for you as far as promoting this device and getting you paid when you use it. If you have any kind of problem even remotely related to the DAC-III or National Medical Innovations, you call me. If you look at the resource page in your packets you'll see my home phone number. Not even my salesmen have that one." There was a snicker from the room. "Don't hesitate to use it — but don't give it to my salesmen."

"In a few days we'll be contacting you to arrange delivery of your equipment. It's yours to use for a year. All we ask is that you follow the protocols and keep accurate records of all the procedures you do. We also ask that you tape the operations from beginning to end and send us a copy of each tape. We want to analyze them just to make sure that everything's working the way it should be."

"You'll also receive your video in about a week. Feel free to show it to any patient who might be a candidate for a DAC-III Sonomagnetic Laser Endometrial Ablation."

There were several more minutes of "thank yous" and "glad you could comes" and then the creaseless sales force dispersed around the room and presented elaborate, very official looking certificates to each of the participants. Dackel read his. Along with the date and a lot of signatures, it said,

This is to Certify that
Alfred Dackel, M.D.
Has Successfully Completed an Approved
Didactic and Hands-On Course
On Hysteroscopic Endometrial Ablation
Using the DAC-III Sonomagnetic Laser

That's a joke, Dackel thought. I hang this on my wall and everybody thinks I know what I'm doing.

Everyone except Dackel walked out to the bus to go back to the hotel. Dackel had his car and besides he wanted to call Carrie to see how she was. He let the phone ring twenty times. He knew after the first five that there would be no answer. He hoped she was all right. He crumpled her phone number and threw it in the trash basket. He couldn't wait to see Red's reaction when he tells him that a naked stripper asked him to spend the night and he refused, and then he threw away her number. He didn't think he would be able to disagree with anything that Red would call him.

On his way back to the car he passed Donny Moline carrying a stack of videotapes.

"Good job, Dr. Dackel. I was watching from the control room."

Dackel nodded and drove back to the hotel. He didn't want to be bothered with returning the car, so he called Avis, and told them it wouldn't start and he refused to pay for the last day. He took the hotel shuttle to the airport.

Chapter 12

Dackel got to the terminal an hour before his flight and he started to become anxious. He went to the bar and had a couple of drinks. He was sitting in a big leather chair in the lounge when he awoke with a start and realized that his flight was scheduled to leave in four minutes. Fortunately, it was ten minutes behind schedule, so he made it just in time. As he was about to sit down in his seat, he noticed a wallet on the floor. He picked it up and opened it. The first thing he saw was a badge. It said "private investigator." He flipped over the leather flap to which it was attached and saw that it belonged to a Bruce Cosmo. The next thing he saw was that the wallet contained about six thousand dollars in hundreds. He rang for the cabin attendant and was about to give her the wallet, but he changed his mind. For some reason he didn't trust her. He wasn't sure why. He asked for a drink of water and put the wallet in his pocket.

The plane landed in Philadelphia with a bigger bump than usual. It woke Dackel from a sound sleep. He felt fuzzy and stiff and generally terrible. As soon as he got into the terminal he called the number in the wallet.

"Answering service"

"Is this Bruce Cosmo's answering service?"

"Yes it is."

"Can you give me Mr. Cosmo's home number?"

"Sorry sir, we're not permitted to do that."

"Well, will you give him the message that I found his wallet and I'll Fed-Ex it back to him in the morning. My name is Dr. Alfred Dackel and my phone number is 215 555-2306."

He drove home expecting to find his dinner waiting. Instead there was a note on the door.

Squirrel is still in the house.
Took the dog and went to my sister's.
I don't want her to get rabies.
Terminix will be here tomorrow.
Shoshi

When she turned fifty Arlene legally changed her name to Shoshana because she felt that "Arlene" wasn't exotic enough. She insisted that everyone call her Shoshi. She changed it back when someone at her aerobics class asked her if she was of Japanese extraction, but she still used it once in a while. Lately she had been considering changing it again by moving the "e" in "Arlene" and making it "Arleen."

"For Christ Sakes," he muttered out loud. He opened the door and before he even turned on the light, a ball of gray fur ran right between his legs and scampered up the large English sycamore. He went to the phone and called his sister-in-law's house.

"Yuh," his brother-in-law answered when he picked up the phone. Lou talked mostly in monosyllabic sounds, most of which you really couldn't call words.

"Hi Lou, it's Al. Arlene there?"

"Yuh," Lou answered, and that's all he answered.

A few seconds later Arlene could be heard in the background.

"Where's he calling from Lou? Is he home Lou? I left a message for him yesterday but he never called me back." Her voice got gradually louder and more piercing as she got closer to the phone.

"Al," she said, louder than she needed to, "where are you, Al? Are you home or are you still in Texas?"

"Florida," he corrected, shaking his head, "I was in Florida, but now I'm home. Come on home."

"Al, there's a squirrel in the house, Al. I'm not coming home until the exterminator gets the squirrel out of the house. He's coming tomorrow, in the morning. I'll come home to let him in, but..."

"The squirrel's gone Arlene."

"How do you know the squirrel's gone Al, maybe he's sleeping or hiding somewhere. Just because you don't see him doesn't mean..."

"Arlene, the squirrel's gone. I saw him run out of the house when I opened the door."

"Al, are you sure he's gone Al? Because..."

"The squirrel's gone Arlene. Come home."

"We're just sitting down to dinner, Al. why don't you come over here because we just sat down to dinner. Rita made..."

"Arlene, I'm tired and I need a shower. You stay for dinner and then come home. I'll find something."

"There's leftover spinach lasagna. It's no-fat. And there's also some no-fat cottage cheese with cinnamon and apples or maybe it's the one with strawberries, I'm not sure which one is left because I ate one yesterday and I don't remember..."

"I'll be fine Arlene. Just eat your dinner and come home. I'll see you soon. Bye."

He hung up before she could start another mini-series.

Al was asleep by the time she got home. He had eaten the cottage cheese (with strawberries), showered and conked out with the light still on. When Arlene came in she kissed him on the head, got into her nightgown and got into bed with her latest Danielle Steele.

Chapter 13

At 6:20 AM Monday morning Dackel awoke to Howard Stern, His favorite morning radio host, berating His producer Baba Booey, for not being able to read his mind. He turned off the clock radio and jumped out of bed. One thing about Dackel was that when he woke up—he was up. It was kind of a necessity in his business. He wasn't looking forward to this day. It was always hard coming back after a weekend away. First he had to see if any of his patients were in labor or if any had delivered. He would call on the way to the office. Then, when he got to the office, there would be a list of his patients who were referred to his coverage, and finally there would be a list of those patients who decided to wait until their doctor got back to town rather than talking to the doctor on call.

He showered and dressed and before he left he kissed Arlene on her head, almost the same way she kissed him the night before. He called Gene Porter from the car and found out that no one was in labor, but Gene had delivered a patient of his on Saturday afternoon. She was home already, of course, because QHM required that she leave the hospital within 24 hours of the delivery unless she had a complication. She was the only QHM patient that they had allowed to stay with him after he got kicked out. They wanted her to transfer but she threatened to sue. The irony is that had she transferred, it would have been to Porter's practice.

He got to the office and made a note to call the newest mother in his practice. He filled out a Fed Ex slip, put the wallet into an envelope and sealed it himself. He would have his secretary drop it in the box when she went to the bank. He looked at his schedule. It wasn't as bad as he thought. He looked down the list and didn't see any of his crazies and didn't even see anyone he didn't like. He had fourteen patients scheduled between 8 and 12 o'clock, and 13 from 1 to 4. Dackel liked to allow a half-hour for new patients and 15 minutes for routine annuals. QHM once sent a memo suggesting that he should be able to see 8 to 12 patients an hour.

At five he had an appointment with a psychiatrist by the name of Dr. Carlton Capuston. He wasn't sure he was going to keep it. It was part of one of Red's harebrained schemes that Al really didn't want to go along with, but from the time they were kids, Dackel generally did whatever Red told him to do.

The day was fairly routine, mostly annual check-ups, a few vaginal itches, a pelvic pain and one woman with a vaginal odor. The odor turned out to be from a tampon that she had forgotten to remove after her last period which had been over for three weeks. The story was typical. Her chief complaint was an odor "like something died in there." They all said that. They also all complained of a watery brownish discharge. He could usually make the diagnosis just by the history. Inhaling usually confirmed it. He asked her a few routine questions, although the answers rarely mattered for this particular problem.

"Is it possible that you left a tampon in?"

"Of course not!" she answered as everyone always does. In fact, it was interesting that every once in a while, someone comes in thinking they had left one in, and it usually turns out that they hadn't, but the ones with the brown discharge and the "something died" smell, you could bet your lunch that they harbored a forgotten tampon.

Whenever he came across this particular situation he implemented his "something died in there" attack plan. He put her in his least favorite examining room and prepared to retire that room for the day. He prepared a plastic urine specimen container by filling it one third of the way with Betadine, an antiseptic iodine solution that kills germs faster than Listerine (or so he was led to believe), and he put on two pairs of latex gloves.

If his patient needed her blood pressure checked or her breasts examined, he did that first. Then he laid out a long forceps, the plastic container with the Betadine and a speculum, and in almost one motion he inserted the speculum, grasped the fetid lump of brown, old blood soaked synthetic fiber, plunged it into the jar and screwed on the lid tightly, all the time holding his breath. The extra pair of gloves was in case he had to touch it for some reason. If he did, he would hold the tampon in his palm and take off the top glove turning it inside out as he took it off. He would then twist the cuff end of the glove and stuff the whole thing into the jar. He had fine-tuned this maneuver over the years and had gotten his time down to under four seconds. Few could do it faster.

He only had one disaster and that was before the days of the Occupational Safety and Health Administration (OSHA) requirement that anything contaminated with bodily fluids had to be put into a special medical waste container. He had thrown the jar into a regular trashcan, and one of his nurses had stomped it down with her foot later that afternoon. The jar broke. He closed down early that day.

That was the only good thing OSHA had ever done for him. He couldn't figure out why a woman could throw a sanitary napkin in the trash in a rest room or a man could toss a condom in the waste basket in his home, but doctors had to pay an approved medical waste company fifty dollars a month to remove Q-Tips that touched the inside of the vagina.

At 10:15 Dackel got buzzed by his secretary. "There's a Mr. Cosmo on the phone," she said.

"Put him through. Hello."

"Hi, is this Dr. Dackel?" asked a man with an accent that sounded more Havana than Tampa.

"Yes, that's me."

"Dr., I got your message last night. I wanted to call and thank you and I'd like to give you something for your effort and your honesty."

"No need," said Dackel, "anyone would have done the same."

"I beg to differ. In my line I see how dishonest people can be. You are an exception and I 'd like to send you a little..."

"No need Mr. Cosmo, you'll have it by tomorrow and it was my pleasure."

"Well, if there's anything I can ever do for you, please call me. I'm based in Tampa, but if you ever need any help, please don't hesitate."

"I'll keep that in mind. Just a word of advice, button your back pocket."

They both laughed, said good-bye and hung up.

The rest of the day was busy but boring. After his last patient left he called Red.

"Hey man, thanks for getting me hooked up with National. The course was really good, but I don't know if I'm ready to do this stuff on my own, I might want to go watch somebody who knows what they're doing for a couple of cases before I try it."

One thing about Dackel, he knew what he didn't know. That was probably the reason he was so apprehensive about trying new things.

"I got you covered," said Red, I already talked to some people from the company. Not that I was checking up on you, I just wanted to see how the first course went."

"What'd they tell you?"

"They said it went fine. They also picked up on the fact that this stuff was pretty new to you but they felt that you did good in the lab and they're sure you'll be able to master the abatin...absolat..."

"Ablation."

"Yeah, whatever. But what's this about you missing one of the labs?"

"Red, it's a long story that's wilder than anything either of us ever made up. I'll tell you when we have some time."

"You got laid!" said Red.

"I didn't get laid."

You ate at the Y, I know it."

"I didn't get laid and I didn't have oral sex," Dackel insisted.

"Then there was no reason for you to have missed the lab."

"I'll tell you about it later. Listen Red, about this psychiatrist thing, I don't know."

"Al, I checked into it. It may be your ticket out of managed care and into semi-retirement paradise. Trust me, it's foolproof."

"But it's not legal."

"Who's to say? If you do this right, there's no way anyone will ever suspect anything, and if they do they'll never be able to prove a thing."

"I just don't know if I can pull it off."

"There's nothing to pull, dickhead. Just do what we discussed. If it doesn't work, it doesn't work. Tell me about the shrink."

"Well he's in his early forties. I got his name from Arnie Geller, one of the anesthesiologists on the staff at Fourteenth Street. Arnie was one of my old students. This guy started out as a physicist. He went to medical school and then became an anesthesiologist. That's when Arnie met him. He didn't like anesthesia so then he did a radiology residency and then went straight to a psychiatry residency. He's only been practicing a few years. From what I gather he's book smart but he has no common sense. His practice is mostly bored housewives, and recently fired middle-aged executives. He doesn't like crazy people and if anybody is really sick, he refers them out."

"Perfect. Just do what we talked about."

"Dr. Dackel," said the voice over the intercom, "its a Ms. Metzger-something on line 2. Should I take a message?"

"No, I'll pick up in a minute."

"Listen, Red, I gotta go. Shoulder pads is on the phone."

"Talk on you later baby," said Red, imitating something he once heard in a Sammy Davis Jr. movie.

"Msssss. Minkman, how are you today?"

"Fiiiine, Dr. Dackel, how was the courrrse," she whined.

How this woman would be able to teach him anything about public speaking was beyond comprehension, but everyone said she was good and he certainly didn't know anyone else in the field. He also realized that he needed some coaching before he did any radio or television interviews.

"It was fine. Your name came up in some literature they gave us. Apparently you're supposed to know what you're doing."

"Oh I do, Dr. Dackel, I do."

"What's the next step?" he asked.

"I want to set up an afternoon when we can prepare for some television and radio interviews."

"I don't have an afternoon, can we do it on the weekend?"

"I try not to work on the weekends but I do have Thursday evening open."

"What time?" he asked.

"7:30. I'll have you out by 10:30."

"Where?"

"My office is on Twelfth Street, not far from yours."

"How much is this going to cost?"

"We'll discuss it on Thursday."

"We'll discuss it now," he said.

"We'll discuss it on Thursday," she said and hung up.

"People who I hire don't hang up on me!" he screamed into the dead receiver, but even while he was yelling, he knew that he would show up. So did she. He admired her toughness and respected her reputation. And for some reason, she, once again, made his penis twitch.

Chapter 14

Carlton Capuston had a small office in a tired looking building just a block away from Dackel's office. It consisted of an embarrassingly tiny waiting room with two inexpensive chairs, a magazine rack with a few old Newsweeks, a ratty National Geographic, and an issue of Games Magazine with all the puzzles already done—in ink. When Dackel arrived, there was no one else in the waiting room. At five on the dot the door to Capuston's office opened and he motioned Dackel into his office.

It, too, was a plain room, barely big enough for a bookcase, a filing cabinet, a small desk with a telephone and a combination fax/copier/printer/answering machine. There were two cheap but comfortable chairs with a small square table between them. On the table was a box of tissues. It made Dackel wonder if he was supposed to cry at some point. He would talk to Red about that later. There was a plant that needed as much attention as Capuston's hair.

"Hello Dr. Dackel, I'm Dr. Carlton Capuston. I don't believe we've ever met," he said with what seemed like a great deal of effort. Capuston was a thin, bony man with a full but scraggly beard and mustache. The mustache seemed to curl around his top lip making it look like he didn't have one. You couldn't see his bottom lip either, but it didn't matter much, because it sounded like he didn't move them a whole lot when he talked. He spoke very, very slowly with a voice that sounded like Kermit the Frog with a mouth full of peanut butter—under water. He spoke so quietly that he gave the impression that his lungs hadn't been fully expanded for some time. He was balding although he had more hair than Dackel. It looked like it had been randomly dropped on his head. He was wearing an out of style, dark plaid shirt that looked like it might have come from the first edition of the L.L. Bean catalog. The collar was buttoned and the elbows were threadbare. Dackel was surprised that there was no pocket protector. He also wore a pair of cotton Dockers, shiny at the knee, and a pair of brown shoes that had obviously never been polished. He smelled like week-old vegetable soup.

"No I don't believe we have met. This is a little uncomfortable for me," said Dackel.

"Me too," said Capuston, "I've never had a doctor as a patient before."

This kid's gonna go far, Dackel thought to himself.

"Why don't you tell me why you're here, Alfred. May I call you Alfred?"

"Sure, can I call you Carlton or Carl?"

"I'd rather you not, under these circumstances."

Under these circumstances? he thought. Under these circumstances I'd be out the door at this point, but he'd promised Red he'd stick to the plan, and that's what he did. For the next forty minutes Dackel told Dr. Capuston about vague feelings of anxiety, trouble sleeping, loss of appetite, decrease in sex drive, feeling overwhelmed, having nothing to look forward to, wishing that the world would stop spinning so fast, and every other cliche he had heard that indicated anxiety or depression. He was careful not to talk about the one thing that Red told him not to.

Capuston sat there, both feet flat on the floor, left hand on left knee, right hand on right. He stared straight at Dackel, glancing down only occasionally to make sure his tape recorder was operating. He had a yellow pad on the table but he took no notes. Nor did he ask any questions. When Dackel finished a thought, Capuston just stared at him until he began another.

At 5:50 he stopped him in the middle of a sentence.

"You'll need to come twice a week. My fee is $135 for a fifty-minute session. I don't believe in professional courtesy. Your insurance may cover part of the fee if you don't mind telling them you're seeing a psychiatrist."

Quite the opposite, Dackel thought, I want them to know.

"Twice a week, is that really necessary? I would prefer once."

"Okay, once will be fine. Is this time satisfactory?"

What a wimp, he thought. "Yes," he said, "this is fine."

He called Red from the car.

"How'd it go?"

"Well, I don't like the idea any better than I did before, but it's going to be easier than I thought."

"Good," said Red, "Don't forget to submit the visits to your insurance company."

"Red, are you sure this thing isn't going to jump up and bite me in the ass?"

"Never happen, old buddy, never happen."

Chapter 15

"I won't be home for dinner Thursday," Al told Arlene over a dinner of grilled vegetables and brown rice.

"Why, where will you be, Al? Do you have a meeting or..."

"I have a meeting with the practice consultant that Red set me up with."

"Al, tell me what's going on, Al. You said something about managed care but what is going on? I know you don't like to talk about business things but I would like to know. Maybe I could help out in the office or something or maybe..."

"Arlene, everything's going to be okay. There were some changes in my situation with one of the insurance companies and this consultant is going to give me some advice. That's all, and I have a meeting with her on Thursday night."

"Her? It's a woman consultant, and you're meeting her at night?"

Arlene Dackel could never decide whether or not her husband ran around on her. She didn't think so because he seemed to so have so little interest in sex, but on the other hand, maybe he just wasn't interested in her. He never really gave her any reason to be suspicious, but it was always in the back of her mind. Red, on the other hand, she was sure Red cheated on his wife. She was wrong.

"Yes, it's a woman and we're meeting at night because I don't have any time during the day. What's for dessert?"

"Low fat apple crisp with no-fat frozen yogurt."

It wasn't bad. When he finished, he read the paper, turned on the television and promptly fell asleep.

The next day his first patient was new to his practice. Her name was Linda Shintock, she was 37 years old, had three children and her tubes had been tied at the time of her last delivery.

"My husband will be up in a minute," she said nervously. "He's parking the car."

Dackel liked it most of the time when the husbands came to the office. They were good to have around in case any decisions had to be made, and often he found that he could explain things better to the husband who would then explain it to his wife. Men were also quicker to choose surgery when there was an option. They seemed to have more of a "do it and get it over with" attitude. Paul Shintock walked in the door just as she finished her sentence.

After the introductions, Dackel asked Linda why she made the appointment.

"I've been bleeding for over a year now. My period's very heavy and it lasts for ten or twelve days. I've been going to a doctor in my neighborhood and she's had me on all different kinds of hormones. I've had two D&C's and during the last one she also did a hysteroscopy. She said she didn't find anything except a few small fibroids and she says I need a hysterectomy. I'm here for a second opinion. I'm not afraid of surgery, it's just that a hysterectomy seems so radical."

"Tell him what you heard, hon," interjected Paul.

"Well," she said blushing, "My neighbor gave me this book that said that after a hysterectomy, you, you know, lose--you lose your, you know..."

Dackel knew. "Your sex drive?" he guessed.

"Yes, that's what she read."

This was something that came up a lot. There were conflicting articles in the literature. Some studies said that sexual desire was affected after hysterectomy, some said it was orgasm that changed, some said that there was no difference and some said sex was better. Dackel read them all but he also had the experience of having done a lot of hysterectomies and seeing the results for himself.

"It depends on the patient," he said. If you're having pain or bleeding before your surgery, and the operation makes it better, then your sex life will probably be better. The same goes for bleeding. If you believe that sex is just for procreation, then you might have some problems with desire once your uterus is out."

"That's not us," she said. "As I mentioned, I had my tubes tied. And you're right, we don't like to have sex when I'm bleeding, so almost half the month is out."

Dackel' s explanation was correct. There was more that he didn't say though, partially because he didn't believe it. There were some articles that talked about different feelings during orgasm when the uterus was removed. Most of these studies were old and not very scientifically grounded, but he had the occasional patient who told him that things were just not the same after the operation.

"But most people tell me that sex is the same as it was before the operation." That was the truth.

He continued to take her history detailing when she got her first period, when it started to become abnormal, the specifics of each of her pregnancies, her previous illnesses and operations, medications she was taking and her allergies. He asked about the health of her parents, her siblings and her children. He questioned her about alcohol and tobacco. If not on the cutting edge of alternative surgery, Al Dackel was very skilled at the basic rudiments of medicine. He always took a thorough history and performed a complete physical examination on every new patient. The problem was he was not the best medical record keeper in the world.

He would go through a series of questions called a "review of systems" during which he would ask, sometimes in one sentence, whether the patient, has had, "any headaches, dizziness, fainting, difficulty hearing, ringing in the ears, discharge from the ears, double vision, blurred vision, sore throats, coughing, coughing up blood, chest pain, shortness of breath, extra heart beats, skipped heart beats, abdominal pain, nausea, vomiting, diarrhea, constipation, blood in the stool, mucous in the stool, rectal itching, burning during urination, frequency of urination, blood in the urine, dark urine, vaginal discharge, itching or burning, vaginal odor, pains in the legs, numbness or tingling in the arms or legs.

If they had any of those problems, he would note them. Occasionally he would note what are called pertinent negatives. For example if a patient had burning during urination, he might note "no blood in urine, no frequency." But if a patient had no complaints, he would write ROS - (review of systems, negative). The insurance carriers, especially Medicare and the managed care companies wanted him to document that he asked all the questions regardless of how the patient answered.

"They want me to see more patients per hour, they want to pay me less, but they want me to spend more time keeping totally unnecessary records," he would complain whenever the opportunity came up.

After taking Linda's history, he escorted her into an examining room. The physical examination was unremarkable, so he wrote "PE -" on her chart. He did feel a tiny fibroid but he felt it was inconsequential and not related to her bleeding. When they returned to his consultation room, he said, "Folks, I want to get copies of the operative and pathology reports from your other doctor. From what you tell me she's done all that can be done hormonally to try to control your bleeding. But there is an—alternative to hysterectomy." He caught himself just as he was about to say '*alterrrnative*.'

"It's called endometrial ablation, Did she talk about that at all?"

"I actually brought it up," replied Linda, "but she said it was still experimental and she didn't feel it was right for me."

"Well it may be right for you and, in a few weeks, I'll be getting a new instrument that will make it safer and more effective than any of the other methods out there. Let me get a copy of your records and I'll call you."

He rose to shake their hands and almost as if he was compelled to turn a perfectly professional, almost classy conversation into something less, he said to Paul, "Don't worry buddy, I'll have you back in the saddle in no time."

Paul smiled. Linda did too, but neither of them seemed all that amused.

Dackel finished his hours at 5 o'clock. He was ten minutes late for the weekly departmental morbidity and mortality conference. This was a meeting mandated by the Quality Assurance Department of his hospital. It was mandated that they mandate it by the Joint Commission on the Accreditation of Hospitals. It was actually a worthwhile meeting for most of the staff. They discussed all of the complications that week that resulted in additional illness (morbidity) or death (mortality). The cases were chosen by the chief resident and usually consisted of patients who developed post-operative fevers or infections. Once a month or so there would be a patient who needed to go back to the operating room, and a few times a year they would have to discuss a death. With the exception of the cancer division, it was rare that anyone died on the obstetrics and gynecology service.

At the meeting they also sometimes discussed questionable management decisions. Two of Dackel's cases were being presented today. His resident rattled off the first history in standard form, way too fast for anyone but another gynecologist to understand.

"This 56 year old white female gravida 3 para 2012 was admitted with a four centimeter left adnexal mass which was complex on ultrasound with a borderline Doppler. CA125 was normal. Admission studies were all normal. She was taken to the O.R. for a TAHBSO. Frozen was benign. EBL was 900 cc's. Post-op course was uneventful and the patient was discharged on the third post-operative day. Final path, benign epithelial cyst. The uterus and other ovary were normal. "

Glossary:

gravida- The total number of times a woman has been pregnant.

para- Results of those pregnancies. The first number stands for full term babies delivered. The second number represents number of premature babies delivered. The third number is the number of miscarriages or abortions, and the last number is the number of living children.

adnexal- Pertaining to the area adjacent to the uterus. Adnexal masses are usually cysts, tumors or swellings of the ovary or fallopian tube.

complex- A mass that is not entirely fluid filled on ultrasound. The complexity usually results from tissue within the cyst, but can also represent blood or debris. Complex masses are more likely to be malignant. Simple or non-complex masses are more likely to be benign.

Doppler- A test done at the same time as the ultrasound that measures blood flow to a mass. The characteristics of the blood flow can often indicate whether a mass is likely to be benign or malignant.

CA125- A blood test that measures a substance that is elevated in about two thirds of women with ovarian cancer. Unfortunately the test is not very specific. It is normal in about one third of ovarian cancers and is elevated in women with many other conditions such as fibroids, endometriosis, infection and about 1% or normal women. The test has been around for a while but was made popular by Gene Wilder after the death of his wife, Gilda Radner. He made some public service announcements urging women to ask their doctors for the test. Unfortunately, because of its non-specificity, many women and doctors panicked. This resulted in many unnecessary operations. It also gave some women a false sense of security when it was negative.

OR- Operating room

TAHBSO Total abdominal hysterectomy, bilateral salpingo-oophorectomy. A total abdominal hysterectomy is removal of the uterus and cervix through an abdominal incision. A bilateral salpingo-oophorectomy is removal of both fallopian tubes and ovaries. Salpingo refers to the tubes, oophor refers to the ovaries. There is a common misconception that total hysterectomy means that the ovaries and tubes are removed. It does not.

Frozen- Frozen section. A frozen section is a microscopic examination of tissue that is usually done while the patient is still on

	the operating table. Its purpose is to allow the surgeon to decide whether additional surgery is indicated, such as in the case of cancer. It is called a frozen section because the pathologist freezes the tissue so it can be cut into thin sections and viewed under the microscope. Normally the tissue is embedded in paraffin to make it easy to cut but that requires more time.
EBL-	Estimated blood loss.
Final path-	Pathologist's interpretation of the tissue after all tests and examinations have been completed.
Benign-	Non-cancerous
Epithelial-	A type of tissue that usually makes up the outer layer of an organ.
Cyst-	A fluid filled tumor.

When he heard the presentation, Dackel was puzzled. The patient did well, she had no complications and she left the hospital in just a few days.

"I bring this case up because I thought that the choice of procedure would make for an interesting discussion," said Dr. Pat Washington, a senior resident who had graduated first in her class from Howard University School of Medicine. "Any comments?"

"Why did you choose to do a hysterectomy, Dr. Dackel?" asked Jimmy Hayes, a second year.

Dackel started to feel threatened. "I chose it because it was the right thing to do," he said defensively. "Suppose the frozen was wrong. Suppose she had cancer. Then I'd have to go back in and take everything out anyway. Why, what would you have done?"

"I would have looked at the ultrasound and seen that even though they called it complex, there was only one questionable septation. Between that, the normal CA125 and a fairly reassuring

Doppler, I would have taken the ovary out laparoscopically and done a frozen."

"Oh you would have, would you?" said Dackel smugly, "And what if it had been malignant, you would have dragged that ovary all over the pelvis before you squeezed it out the tiny incision."

"No sir, I would have put it in a bag."

Dackel had read about plastic bags that could be used for removing tissue laparoscopically, but he had never used one because he didn't do any laparoscopic removal of anything. The bag was collapsed around a stick. Once it was inserted into the abdomen through a small entry port, it was opened and the tissue was placed inside. It was then closed with a drawstring and the mouth of the bag was brought out through the same small incision. Forceps and, if necessary, scissors, were then used to remove the tissue without spilling a drop inside the body.

"Well, I don't believe in that. I do things the way I was taught and it's worked for me for almost thirty years."

"I agree with Dr. Dackel," said Shelby Davis, another senior resident. "If there's any chance of cancer I would prefer to open her up, but I would have trusted the frozen, especially with a negative CA and only a borderline Doppler. I would have stopped at removing the ovary. Maybe I would have removed the other one, but I would have left the uterus."

The chairman of the committee spoke. "You're right Pat, this was an interesting case from a management standpoint, and I want you all to know that you might all be correct, and you might all be wrong.

Jimmy, those bags break with some regularity. If you spilled some cancer you might change her stage. On the other hand, some say that it's okay to spill some cells if you open up right away and irrigate copiously.

Shelby, it might work your way too, but what if the permanent path was different from the frozen? Besides, without her uterus to worry about, it makes it easier for her to take hormone replacement.

Al, according to the operative note, you lost most of that blood taking out the uterus. If you left her uterus in you wouldn't have had the problem. So you see, there are no rules and no guarantees in medicine. The same decision might be right one day and wrong the next."

Dackel felt exonerated, but so did Hayes and Davis. The second case, presented by Dr. Washington, was a 45-year-old patient of Dackel's who had a hysterectomy for excessive bleeding. The operation had gone well. The pathology report showed a normal, uterus, tubes and ovaries. The patient also had some excessive blood loss during the case and required a transfusion of one unit of blood.

Dr. Washington continued, "I bring this case up for two reasons. First, quality assurance kicked it to me to present because there is inadequate documentation in the records of hormonal treatments, D&C's or other attempts to manage the bleeding. They feel that if this case was audited it would be denied by the insurance company. We're all used to Dr. Dackel's documentation techniques, [laughter in the room] but the QA people aren't. More importantly, I presented this case to serve as a jump off point for a discussion about alternative management strategies for dysfunctional uterine bleeding, or for the students in the room, bleeding without a physical or structural cause. Any comments?"

"Did you consider endometrial ablation, Dr. Dackel?" asked someone whose name he didn't know.

"No, I didn't, because at the time I didn't do the procedure. It might interest you to know, however, that in a few weeks, I will be starting to do DAC-III endometrial ablations. What the DAC-III is..."

"Wow, Dr. Dackel, we know what it is," said Pat, "It's been all over the literature and we even discussed it at our last journal club. I didn't know you even did hysteroscopy."

"Well I do now, and I'll be glad to teach you all how to use the machine when it comes."

"Dibs on the first case," said Washington.

The rest of the conference was uneventful. They probably wouldn't bother him again for a few months unless he had a significant complication.

He went home, had dinner and called Red from his study. Arlene left for her "Self-Actualization Through Sculpting" class at the Institute for Self-Actualization, a holdover women's self-help school from the seventies that was housed in a facility that functioned as a daycare center during the day.

"Hey lover boy," said Red leeringly, "so tell me what kept you from that lab on Sunday."

Dackel went through the whole Angel/Carrie escapade, from their meeting in the strip club, to the coffee, to the phone call and the three AM visit.

"And you didn't nail her?"

"Red, what the fuck are you talking about? You know I don't do that stuff."

"Yeah, but who could have resisted that?"

"She's a kid."

"She's a stripper."

"You're a perv."

"Is something wrong with that?"

"Listen Red, I have something more important to talk about. I've been thinking about this psychiatrist thing. I really don't want to do it. It's not right, and the guy gives me the creeps."

"Al, if you don't like him, try another one. I'm telling you, it will pay off. Hey, do you want to play some cards on Thursday?"

"Can't, I have a date with the deviated septum."

"Who?"

"The hyphen lady."

"You know, I never saw her. She can't be as bad as you described."

"She's not really. Actually if she fixed her hair and got off her high horse, she would be a lot more likable."

"You going to try to nail her."

"You're a real putz, you know! Talk to you later."

Wednesday was another office day. Nothing special happened except the computer crashed and his office manager told him that it was because it didn't have enough memory to handle his patient base since it had been reprogrammed to become Y2K capable. He wasn't really sure what that meant, but he understood real well the thirty five hundred dollars it was going to take to make it right.

"Hold off for a day," he said, "let me check with my practice consultant."

Chapter 16

Dackel awoke on Thursday morning a little excited. He hated to admit it but he was looking forward to his meeting with Deborah Metzger-Minkman. He was also excited about the DAC-III. He went out to his car but when he looked at the sky and smelled the air, he decided that he better take the 4X4. Dackel was convinced that by smelling the air, he could predict snow better than the weathermen. Had he turned on the news station that morning rather than listening to Howard Stern trying to talk a nineteen year old out of her blouse, he would have heard that he was right. They predicted four inches.

With some difficulty, he started up his pride and joy, his ten year old Bronco with the moldy upholstery and the rusted out tailgate and he headed for the hospital. He had only one case scheduled that day. He was starting to feel the loss of his QHM patients. The case was a hysterectomy on a 55 year-old, obese, diabetic woman with cancer of the endometrium (the inner lining of the uterus.) It is not unusual for obese diabetics to get endometrial cancer, and once it is diagnosed there is no choice other than hysterectomy. Maybe someday the DAC-III could cure her, but not today.

The case went well. Just as his resident was putting in the last skin staple, the phone rang. It was his office nurse calling to say that one of his patients was in labor.

"That blows my day," he said. "I thought I'd be able to sneak out and go to a movie, but it looks like I'll be baby-sitting upstairs."

Dackel had decided to give up obstetrics, but this QHM thing had screwed things up. Maybe Red's psychiatrist idea was worth trying. The longer he sat in the coffee room in the labor and delivery suite, the more it appealed to him.

His patient was a primagravida, Latin for "first pregnancy." She had been laboring all night and from the progress curve that he carefully graphed each time he examined her, he estimated that she would deliver by five that evening. She was progressing well and he anticipated no complications, but he had learned a long time ago never to take labor for granted. He didn't, and insisted that his patients be electronically monitored during the entire process. Fetal monitors had become popular when he was still in his young aggressive phase, a period that lasted just a few years. He had become comfortable with them and, at least psychologically, dependent on them.

The monitors recorded fetal heart rate and uterine contractions. By looking at how the heart rate varied during the contractions, he was able to determine whether the placenta was supplying enough blood to the baby. He was pretty good at interpreting fetal monitor tracings and managing labor in general, but more importantly, he was there. When Dackel had a patient in labor, if at all possible, he was in the labor room with her the entire time. He didn't especially like it, but he felt it was the right thing to do. When Patel left, it made it almost impossible for him to do obstetrics the way he felt it should be done so he made the decision to give it up as soon as he could afford to.

At exactly 4:52 P.M. Dackel flawlessly and gently guided a beautiful (despite being covered with blood and slime) seven pound two ounce boy into a world that some say is similarly covered.

"Damn." he said to himself, "a boy." Dackel didn't mind delivering boys as long as they were Jewish. This one was not. His reason was simple. Most parents still wanted their baby boys to be circumcised. The Jewish ones usually had it done during a religious ceremony, in the old days, by a rabbi, but in modern times by a circumcision specialist called a mohel. Everyone else expected the obstetrician to make what he Dackel referred to as "the unkindest cut." He hated doing circumcisions. He had to change his clothes and scrub before he went into the nursery and he didn't like when the babies cried. He also thought the operation was unnecessary. His own son had, of course, been circumcised.

That was an example of the paradox of Alfred Dackel. He had so many inconsistencies. He was basically a good honest guy with conservative, almost what you might call old-fashioned values. He did what he thought was right most of the time. His problem was that he was constantly redefining what he considered right. Sometimes he knew deep in his heart that something was right, like alternatives to hysterectomy, but because he was afraid to learn how to do them, he made them "not right." Hyphenated names were not part of the value system with which he grew up, so they too were wrong.

If you had asked him about circumcision ten years ago, he would have told you that it was a good thing. It wasn't until they started to disrupt his day that he started to agree with most of the pediatric and urologic literature that said they were unnecessary.

He finished with the delivery, repaired the episiotomy meticulously and went out to the waiting room to congratulate the anxiously awaiting father and grandparents. Most of the obstetricians at his hospital welcomed fathers into the delivery room, but Dackel did not. He tried it once at a patient's insistence and when he cut the episiotomy, the father passed out and gashed his head. That was the first and last time he allowed a "support person" into the delivery room.

Dackel showered and shaved. He didn't really need a shave that badly, but he was tired and, for some reason, shaving revitalized him. He didn't even consider the possibility that he might have decided to shave for the benefit of one practice consultant with the initials of DM-M. He ate a quick dinner in the hospital cafeteria, passing on the "heart smart " menu and opting instead for a roast pork with provolone on garlic bread. Then, realizing what he had done, he went to the gift shop, bought a pack of Breath Asure and swallowed about ten of them, more than three times the recommended dosage.

He stopped back at his office and went through his mail. There was a letter from National Medical Innovations thanking him for coming to the course and advising him that the DAC-III unit would be shipped on February 9th. He felt a little anxious when he realized that it was less than a month away. They also informed him that the company had gotten full FDA approval to start the phase two testing and that he could start to schedule patients at any time. Because they knew whom they were dealing with, the letter also said that Dr. Mark MacDonald himself would like to be present during Dackel's first case.

"Thank God," he said out loud. The ablation looked easy enough, but there was a lot of equipment. Besides, he missed the Sunday lab and he had still never performed a basic hysteroscopy on a real person.

There was also an envelope with Linda Shintock's records from her other gynecologist.

Boy that was fast, he said to himself. I don't think my office responds to records requests that quickly.

The records reflected pretty much what Linda had said. She had been bleeding long and heavily for about a year and a half. She had been tried on three or four different hormones without success and she had two D&C's neither showing any good reason for her bleeding, and neither solving her problem. There were copies of pictures taken during her hysteroscopy but the poor reproductions together with Dackel's inexperience with interpreting what he was looking at made them essentially useless. The doctors notes revealed her frustration with Linda's problem. The last one said,

"Discussed with pt. See no choice at this point other than hysterectomy. Pt asked about alternatives. Advised experimental. Suggested second opinion. Meanwhile, given Depo-Lupron."

Lupron was one of a relatively new class of drugs that threw women into an artificial menopause. It was also one of the medications that was used to shrink the lining of the uterus prior to endometrial ablation.

From what Dackel could gather, Linda Shintock looked like a perfect candidate for DAC-III Sonomagnetic Endometrial Ablation, or whatever they called it. He left a note for his secretary to call the Shintocks and set up another appointment.

Dackel picked up two phone messages that were on the corner of his desk where his secretary always put them. One was from Red. There was almost always one from Red. The other was from Carrie Bradford. He dialed her number but there was no answer. He hoped everything was okay. He would call back later.

He arrived at Deborah Metzger-Minkman's office at ten minutes to seven. The office was nothing special, but he thought Metzger-Minkman looked pretty good despite the fact that 30-40% of her left upper incisor was smudged with lipstick and her hair had somehow gotten frizzier. He wondered for a moment, whether there was a chance she made it look that way on purpose, although he seriously doubted that anyone would. She was wearing a short black skirt and a v-neck pink angora sweater which showed more cleavage than she intended.

"Hiiiii Doctor Daaackel," she whined.

Real estate, he thought, or an interior decorator, or even a jewelry store sales person. But a medical practice consultant and a media trainer? Who is she kidding?

"Are you ready to get starrrted?"

"You said we'd discuss fees tonight," he answered.

"Oh yes," she remembered. "I charge a hundred and fifty dollars an hour for media coaching. I figure you'll need about twelve to fifteen hours, so that part will be between $3000 and $3750. But I also want to go over your billing and collection system, your fees schedule, your insurance company contracts and your personnel policies and..."

"How much?"

"Including the media training and placements and everything else, I figure ten grand will cover it."

"Good-bye, Ms. Minkman, it's been nice."

"Wait a minute," Dr. Dackel, "hear me out. Your gross income last year was four hundred and ninety six thousand dollars. Mr. Klee estimates that without the QHM income, this year you'll gross three thirty. We'll split the difference. You don't pay me one cent until you bring in four hundred and thirteen thousand dollars. If you make one penny less, you owe me nothing."

The math didn't sound right but he didn't feel like figuring it out so he just pretended that he was. After a few seconds he looked up and nodded his head.

"Okay, but when do I get to call you Debbie?" he said smiling in an attempt to show her that he changed his mood as well as his mind.

"Probably never," she snapped with absolutely no humor whatsoever in her voice or on her face. "Let's get started. First I want you to watch this tape of a Bob Newhart show..."

"Where he gets invited to be a guest on the morning talk show and he screws up," he interrupted.

"Dr. Dackel, how did you know?"

"I'm psychic. Can we move on at a hundred and fifty bucks an hour?"

"Oh, they must have played it at the courrrse."

"Yeah, it must be one of the ABC's of media training."

"No, I think Newhart was on CBS," she smiled and winked. So we'll skip the tape and get to your message."

"You mean my cannon?"

"Oh, now I get it. Dave Evans must have taught a course at your workshop. He's the 'fire the cannon' guy. You can call it that if you want. Other people call it 'planting your flag,' 'lowering your boom,' 'dropping your load,' or one that I don't even like to say."

"Shooting your wad?"

"Dr. Dackel, how did you know that?"

"I told you, I'm psychic. Actually, I guessed, and don't be offended. That's a Civil War term for firing a musket." (He made that up but figured it might be true.)

"Well anyway, what is your message?"

"My message is that I can offer a new alternative to hysterectomy."

"Good," she said, "but let's glitz it up a bit. Aren't you the only doctor in the area offering the new operation? What's it called again?"

"Endometrial Ablation, and I'm not the only one offering it. I'm the only one offering it with the new machine."

"Then let's hit that hard. What's the advantage of the new machine?"

"Over the other methods of endometrial ablation? I don't remember. It has something to do with the device identifying and then targeting only the bad tissue."

"I'll tell you what," she said, "If you give me the literature you got, I'll go through it and come up with what we call copy points, or what Dave Evans calls cannon balls. For now let's practice some basic interview techniques. Suppose a host tries to get you off the subject, for example, suppose she or he asks you how you feel about abortion."

She or he? he said to himself. Did she say she or he? What the hell is that? Who the hell says she or he?

"Dr. Dackel, did you hear me?

Yeah, I heard you. "I would tell him—or her, that abortion is not only a constitutional right, it is a decision that a woman and her doctor should make without the interference..."

"Whoa, hold up. That's the last thing you want to do. You didn't come on the show to talk about abortion. Besides, regardless of which side you take, no one ever wins an abortion debate."

Dackel thought back to the course when Evans asked one of the doctors about fees. He remembered the bridge.

"Okay, how about, 'I'm not here to talk about abortion, I came on the show to talk about alternatives to hysterectomy.'"

"That's the right idea but you have to soften it. You never want to look like you're arguing and you never want to lose your cool. How about if you said, 'Oh, that's an interesting question but it's a topic for another show. Today I want to be sure that I have enough time to tell you and your audience about a new, cutting edge, state of the art procedure that can help a woman

A V O I D   A   H Y S T E R E C T O M Y.'

Did you notice how slowly I said 'avoid a hysterectomy,' and how I emphasized it? That's your cannonball or your flag or your load."

"Or my wad," he said smiling.

She ignored him. "Dr. Dackel, If you do this right, you'll have more patients than you'll know what to do with."

"Before managed care, I did," he said.

"I'm afraid managed care is here to stay," she said. "Isn't it interesting that this all started because Hillary Clinton said she was going to reform health care. She never did it. The managed care explosion was in full swing before one law was proposed, even before one report was issued."

He thought about QHM and ninety thousand dollars a year. He thought about having to learn all this new stuff. He thought about the other participants at the meeting and how energetic and bright they appeared, and how they seemed to catch on to the techniques right away.

"Where'd you go Dr. Daaackel?" Deborah asked in her annoying sing-songy voice, while craning her neck to try to make eye contact with him. "Let's try again. Suppose an interviewer asks you whether alternatives are really better than traditional hysterectomy, or whether all these new things are just gimmicks."

"Do I have to tell the truth?" he asked.

"Come on, Dr. Dackel, what's your message?"

Dackel thought for a few seconds and then slumped down in his chair.

"My message Deborah, is that I feel like a fraud. I know I'm supposed to say that I can offer a new alternative to hysterectomy, using hysteroscopic laser something or other, but the truth is, I don't know how to do the operation. They're even going to send a baby sitter down to help me do my first one."

There was silence for a long time. A concerned look slowly spread from her eyes to the rest of her face. "Al, let me tell you what your problem is. You're frightened. I'm not sure why, but I see it in your eyes and I hear it in your words. I think you're so blustery and angry all the time because the world is changing and you're afraid to change with it. I like you Al. I think you're probably a great doctor and I have a feeling that under all your cantankerousness, you're a good person. Don't ask me how I know. I can just tell." The edge had left her voice. It became softer and almost nurturing.

"You're afraid you won't be able to do the new operations as well as you do the old ones. It's okay to be afraid, but Al, you have to move on. You have to try."

He just sat there. She was right. He knew how to do what he knew how to do and he was afraid of screwing up if he tried something different. He came back from the course excited but now he was petrified.

"Al, I believe in you. National will teach you how to be competent, I'll teach you to be confident. With that combination, you can't lose."

They talked for another half-hour, not about media training, or business, but about life. She confided that her husband had been killed by a mugger eight years ago when her daughter Emma was an infant. He told her that he was happily married, but there was a certain passion missing from his life. She told him that she hadn't had the desire to date since her husband died. He told her that he felt that with all the new technology, his profession was passing him by. She told him that she knew he could learn it and that she would support him.

Finally she stood and told him that she had enjoyed their conversation. They scheduled another meeting for the same time next week. She said, "Good-bye Al, you're a good guy."

He felt like she was hugging him with her voice. He wished she would really hug him. She didn't.

"See you next week."

Dackel went back to his office and checked his messages again. A patient's dog ate her birth control pills and she needed another pack. Mrs. Fink called about her rectal itch. She called three or four times a month about her rectal itch. A new patient, Vivica Bomstein, needed to make an urgent appointment because she "felt weird." He returned all the calls and then dialed Carrie's number.

"Yeah." a woman answered. She sounded too hard to be Carrie.

"Carrie Bradford please."

"Oh, Dr. Dackel," the voice said changing to the one he remembered, "thank you so much for calling. I wouldn't have bothered you but I'm at the end of my rope."

"That's okay Carrie, I was wondering how you were making out."

"Not so well. He came back and beat me up again, Dr. Dackel," she started crying. "I called a lawyer and he wants three hundred dollars to file a restraining order. Dr. Dackel, I don't have a cent. The last time he came he took all my money."

Dackel thought it was strange that she needed a lawyer for a restraining order, but he didn't know Florida law.

"What about the job at the club?" he asked, knowing that she could earn three hundred dollars in an hour or two.

She started to cry. "He- came- in- and- made- a -big scene- and they -fired me," she said, sobbing between almost every word.

"Carrie, I like you a lot but I can't give you three hundred dollars. I just can't."

"That's okay, Dr. Dackel, it was wrong of me to even ask. I'm sorry," she said as she broke into what was now a hysterical cry. "I don't want to be a burden on anyone, it's just not worth it. I can't take it any more."

Dackel recognized the words. He had heard them once before from a patient who wound up swallowing a whole bottle of Xanax and drinking a fifth of vodka. She didn't die, but he learned to be a little more tuned in to suicidal talk.

"Carrie, are you going to do anything to hurt yourself?"

"What's the difference, either I kill myself or he kills me." she said, with a little more composure and what sounded like a lot more commitment.

"Carrie, I want you to go to a hospital tonight. Tell them what you told me. They'll take care of you."

"I don't have any insurance."

"Well how about a friend?"

"He'll find me Dr. Dackel. That's okay, thanks anyway."

"Carrie, make me a promise. If I send you the money, will you promise not to hurt yourself, and to stay with a friend until you can get the restraining order?"

He couldn't hear the answer through her convulsive crying. Finally, he heard her say "yes."

"What's you address, I'll send it right out."

"Don't send it to my apartment. If he finds it, he'll take it. Could you please wire it?"

"I've never wired money before, Carrie, how do I do it?"

She explained how to wire the money via Western Union. She thanked him profusely and hung up. He wired the money and, for the first time in a while, he felt good about himself. After all, he'd blown three hundred bucks on things that were a lot less important.

Dackel got home about ten. Arlene was in bed, reading.

"Arlene, we need to talk. I'm learning some things about myself that I want to share with you."

"Al, what could you possibly learn that you already don't know about yourself, a man your age knows..."

"Arlene, I feel like my profession is passing me by. I'm still practicing like I did the year I finished my residency."

"Al, don't be ridiculous, you're a wonderful doctor, You're fine. There's no need to feel that you're not the best doctor in the hospital. All of the girls at the beauty shop brag about how you..."

"Arlene, I really mean it, I feel like..."

"Don't be ridiculous Al, I don't want to hear another word about this, now come to bed."

"But I..."

"But I, but you. Hush up and come to bed."

"I'll be up soon," he said, with a sincere disappointment in his voice that went right by her, "I'm going downstairs for a few minutes."

"Oh Al, how did your meeting go?"

"Fine, just fine," he said as he left the room and shut the door.

As Dackel walked down the stairs he got the undeniable burning in his eyes that told him that his seldom used tear ducts were going to get their second workout in fifteen years. They did. He cried for an hour before he fell asleep in his recliner.

Chapter 17

Dackel got to his office on Friday morning at about 8, just as the Federal Express early delivery truck drove up. The package contained the video tape that he made in Tampa. He put it into the VCR in his consultation room and pushed play. The tape opened with elaborate graphics over the title "Endometrial Ablation with the DAC-III Sonomagnetic Laser as Performed by Alfred Dackel, M.D." The opening scene was Dackel at the desk in the borrowed shirt and with a pancaked face, which he had to admit, looked pretty good.

"Hello, I'm Dr. Alfred Dackel, and I want you to meet a good friend of mine, Dr. Mark MacDonald, the Medical Director of National Medical Innovations, the company that developed and manufactures the DAC-III. Dr. MacDonald will explain how this unique and wonderful instrument will help me when I perform your endometrial ablation surgery."

The tape then cut to a segment where MacDonald explained the DAC-III procedure in lay terms.

"Hello, I'm Mark MacDonald and I'm going to be your guide for the next few minutes as we watch your doctor perform an endometrial ablation procedure with the DAC-III Sonomagnetic Laser."

After his explanation, the scene then changed to an operating room complete with an anesthesiologist, two nurses, a scrub nurse standing at the operating table and a circulating nurse whose job in a real O.R. is to gather instruments, keep records of how many sponges are used, answer the telephone and operate any non-sterile equipment. In this tape she just stood by the DAC-III and gestured toward it like the models at the car shows. The tape then showed a smiling patient, with perfectly applied lipstick and eye make-up, dressed in a gown and paper cap. She moved from a transport stretcher to the operating table, smiling the whole time.

Then, through the magic of computer editing, Dackel saw himself in that same operating room, dressed in a scrub suit, cap and mask. He saw himself sit down at the foot of the table and appear to put a speculum into the patient's vagina, which was draped so that you couldn't really see that it was a plastic mannequin. It then showed him inserting the hysteroscope. All the time, Dr. MacDonald was narrating.

"As you can see, your doctor is gently inserting the speculum and carefully grasping the cervix or the opening to the womb, with a non-traumatic instrument called a tenaculum."

If they had showed the tenaculum, which really did look like iceman's tongs, the non-traumatic part might not have been very convincing.

"Now you can see how the fluid flows through the hysteroscope to distend the cavity of the uterus."

The video switched to an animation illustrating how the endometrial cavity expands like a balloon when the fluid flows in. It then cut back to Dackel looking like he knew what he was doing.

"Watch as your doctor activates the ultrasound, laser and MRI scans, and look at the monitor as the DAC-III draws a three dimensional map of the pelvic organs and tissues."

The video cut to the monitor and the same example that they had shown during the class.

"Now your doctor will activate the treatment cycle. Watch as the endometrium starts to turn color." They cut to an actual picture of the inside of the uterus. Neither blood nor anything else disgusting was visible. Every five seconds or so it would cut back to Dackel sitting between the mannequin's legs, looking like he was in total control.

"When the operation is over, you'll relax in the recovery room for an hour or so and then you'll be on your way home to rest comfortably for a day in your own bed." The tape showed the patient sitting up in a brass bed wearing a pink peignoir and a pink ribbon in her hair, and covered with a beautiful fluffy down comforter. Of course, she was still smiling and her distinguished gray haired good looking husband was standing over her smiling right back.

"Pretty impressive," he thought to himself. Then he thought about how bogus the whole thing was and how incompetent he was, but then he thought about his talk with Deborah. She was perceptive, and very nice, and she believed in him—and she listened.

His hours usually started at nine, but he had come in early to see Vivica Bomstein, the new patient he had spoken to the night before. She had not been specific about her problem, but she sounded like she really needed to be seen so he agreed to see her at 8:30. It was 8:55 when she walked in, carrying a cup of Dunkin' Donuts coffee.

"Hope you don't mind, I stopped for coffee. I'm nowhere without my coffee in the morning and Dunkin' Donuts has the best."

No "sorry I'm late," no "thank you for seeing me at the last minute," no "thanks for coming in early for me." He already knew he didn't like her. She was early forties, dressed in denim from head to toes including a huge denim pocketbook and even a denim ring that had probably been made out of a belt loop. But it wasn't old, comfortable denim, it was brand new, stiff, denim dyed to look worn. She wore yards and yards of denim, more clothes than Arlene and Metzger-Minkman combined. She looked like she got caught in the middle of an explosion at the Wrangler plant.

He invited her back to his consultation room fully expecting to learn to dislike this woman even more than he already did.

"Can I take my coffee with me?" she asked.

"Sure," answered Dackel's receptionist, earning from him one of his famous "don't ever do that again" stares.

"I need to use the ladies room first, do you need a sample?"

Dackel used to test everyone's urine, but some of the insurers stopped paying for routine urinalyses, so now he only checked urine when he felt it was indicated.

"Are you having any urinary problems?" he asked.

"Oh yes, I have chronic urethritis, interstitial cystitis and a small bladder capacity. I've also had blood in my urine, kidney stones and..."

"Yes, give me a sample, I'll get all the information when you're finished." He knew he was in for a long day.

When she finally came into the consultation room at 9:10, she put her coffee on his desk and then proceeded to knock it over with one of her massive sleeves. It soaked a chart, his Daytimer and the box from his new videocassette.

"Whoops," she said and smiled.

Not "sorry," not "where can I get a towel," just "whoops."

He took a wad of tissues and blotted it up as well as he could.

"How can I help you?" he asked.

"I just don't feel right," she said.

"You need to be more specific Vivica, what doesn't feel right?"

"I don't know if it's my hypoglycemia, or my systemic yeast or my environmental allergies, or maybe it's my chronic fatigue acting up, but I just don't feel right."

Maybe she's allergic to denim, he thought, but instead he asked "Does anything hurt?"

"My joints ache un*bear*ably, but they always do. It's from my fibromyalgia, and I'm in horrible, horrible constant ex*cru*tiating pain from my endometriosis, but no one's been able to do anything about that for 20 years. I've been operated on nine times. I also have horrible ex*cru*tiating pains in my jaw and my neck, but that's TMJ. I wear an appliance at night and I do exercises by putting the tip of my tongue way back on my uppah pahlah lih dhi."

"What?"

"I'm sorry, I said I do exercises by putting the tip of my tongue way back on my upper palate like this." She opened her mouth and flipped her tongue back towards her throat revealing the ugly blue veins on the underside of what just may be the ugliest part of the human body.

"I'm a gynecologist, Ms. Bomstein, how can I help you?"

"I just don't feel right?"

"What doesn't feel right?"

"I don't really know."

Dackel had encountered this type of patient before. It was almost like veterinary medicine. You had to figure out what was going on with very little help from the patient. He took the rest of the history in detail, and she responded positively to almost every question. Did she have chest pain? Sometimes. Did she ever faint? Yes. Did she ever have migraines? Of course. He almost asked her if her hair ever hurt, just to see what she would say, but he didn't.

He examined her and found nothing. He suggested that she have blood taken for a screening test that checked for just about everything, but she refused. He used to feel frustrated when he came across a patient like this, but it didn't bother him anymore. He just resigned himself to the fact that he would probably not be able to help Ms. Bomstein and her kind. He considered them magazine hypochondriacs. Whatever the new fad illness was, they had it. But he also knew that these were the most difficult patients to treat because it was so hard to tell when they were really sick. He felt these pathetic people were attracted to the trendy diseases because their symptoms were so vague. Most of the magazine diseases have just about the same symptoms. Occasionally, though, he would find one who had a thyroid problem or lupus, or some other disease that can give you trendy disease symptoms.

He reassured Vivica that he found nothing wrong with her from a gynecologic perspective, and he advised her to contact her family doctor, her herbalist, her reflexologist and her chiropractor to see if any of them could find a reason for her weird feelings.

It was 9:35. He was already more than a half-hour behind. His next patient was Susan O'Rourke. He'd been taking care of Susan for years. She was about fifty, obese and dirty looking. She had on bright red lipstick, way too much eye shadow and a big floppy hat. Her dress reminded him of the talking parrots in the Tiki Tiki Bird exhibit at Disney World. He could tell by the way she constantly licked her lips and moved her tongue around that she was suffering from dry mouth, probably a result of high doses of psychiatric medications that he she was on.

"How are you today Susie?" he asked."

"Not so good Doc. They kicked me out of the halfway house. One of those managed care things took over taking care of us nuts and they say I'm able to be on my own."

"Susie, you're not nuts. You have a chemical imbalance in your brain and you can't help it. When you take your medicine, you're as normal as I am." That wasn't entirely true, but the first part of his statement was. Susan didn't have any gynecologic complaints. She just needed a routine check up and a Pap smear. Unfortunately, Medicare paid for only one routine Pap every three years, so Dackel was forced to lie and say that it wasn't routine. "Cervical erosion," he wrote on the slip. You'd think the government would be wise to this by now, he thought.

For an impatient man, Dackel had almost unlimited patience for Susan. He felt sorry for her and he liked her. He had lent her a few dollars over the years. Once, she mentioned in conversation that she had never been to a Broadway type show. When the musical Cats came to town he bought her a ticket and sent it anonymously. She knew whom it was from, but neither of them ever mentioned it.

The rest of the day was fairly routine. Mostly just annual check-ups, a few problems here and there, and, oh yes, his clean patient. Everyone has one or two “clean patients,” but Dackel’s was probably the cleanest. She came in once or twice a month just to make sure she didn’t have a vaginal infection. That wasn’t so unusual, but she brought her own speculum. She had purchased it years ago at a women’s health awareness seminar. She didn’t trust that the speculums in any doctor’s office were clean enough for her. Even after Dackel’s nurse showed her the steam sterilizer they used, she still didn’t trust it. She always brought her own in a plastic Zip-Lock bag. She had a few other clean idiosyncrasies. She didn’t like to handle money. She went to the bank weekly to get brand new bills and she made sure she had enough of each denomination so she wouldn’t need change. She couldn’t ask for new coins at the bank, so she would have the teller put the coins in a Zip-Lock bag. When she got home she would transfer them to a mesh bag like the kind used for laundering lingerie. She would then run them through the dishwasher on the extra dirty pot cycle. Dackel had tried many times to talk her into seeking psychiatric care, but she didn’t really perceive that she had a problem, and actually, she functioned very well on the bench of the Pennsylvania State Appellate Court.

Dackel finished early, went over to Red’s office and talked about nothing in particular for a few hours before they both went home to dinner.

The weekend was uneventful. The Dackels attended the wedding of a distant cousin on Saturday night. They actually missed the ceremony because Arlene decided to change her outfit at the last minute because of something about her stockings. They danced twice. He ate three desserts. They got home late and considered having sex, but they both decided they were too tired.

On Sunday he had to go in to deliver a patient. It went well and he was home by a little after noon, but he decided, again, that he was going to give up delivering babies as soon as he possibly could. Of course he had been saying that after every delivery for the last ten years.

Monday the whole thing started again. He finished his schedule, and went straight to Capustan’s office for his second visit. Red had coached him on what to say. Dackel still didn’t like the whole idea.

“How are you Dr. Dackel,” Capuston asked with what seemed like great effort. Dackel put out his hand but Capuston didn’t respond. He was wearing the same clothes as last time and smelled like the vegetable soup had aged another week.

"I'm not too bad today. It seems I have most of my problems the night before surgery."

"Tell me about your childhood, Alfred. "Were you close with your family?"

He hadn't taken the bait. Dackel decided to try the bridge technique that he had learned in his media training class.

"My childhood was pretty normal, but lately I've been getting so uptight whenever I operate."

"Did you have a close relationship with your grandparents?"

"So much for media training," he thought, and then he decided to try again with the hook.

"My grandparents were fine, but I think I know what might be bothering me."

"Um hmm."

Red had told Dackel to let the doctor come to the conclusion by himself, but it was obvious that it wasn't going to happen.

"I think I'm becoming afraid of operating."

Dackel just looked at him waiting for a response. While waiting he looked around the room and started reading all of Capuston's diplomas. He wasn't quite sure, and he hoped he was wrong, but he thought that, out of the corner of his eye, he saw Capuston pick some wax out of ear and put it into his mouth.

"Dr. Capuston, I said I think I'm becoming afraid of doing surgery."

"I heard you," said Capuston, seeming almost frazzled and unsure of where to go next.

Dackel took charge. "It's been going on for a year or so. Every time I go into the O.R., I get nervous." Red had told him not to say any more than that.

"Maybe you shouldn't do any more surgery until you feel better about it. Now why don't we talk about your childhood," Capuston repeated.

Dackel sighed and started to talk about his days at Fifth and Tasker.

Chapter 18

Red knew a guy who knew a guy who was owed a favor by a guy named Spencer Dishay, one of the hundreds of middle level managers that they called vice-presidents at QHM. He arranged a meeting with Dishay on Tuesday afternoon. Red and Dackel met at QHM headquarters in a suburb of Philadelphia.

"Mr. Klee told me of your predicament, Dr. Dackel, and I took the liberty of pulling your file earlier today. It looks like our Mr. O'Brien had somewhat of a hissy fit," Dishay said, winking at Red.

Red smiled, Dackel just shook his head and shrugged his shoulders. "I don't know what I did. We were talking about the new contract and the next thing I knew, he got upset because I didn't dot every i and cross a few t's."

"All's I know," said Red, " is that this doctor's been one of your best health care providers since you guys opened your doors, and it'd be a shame to lose him because of a misunderstanding."

"I can see your point, Mr. Klee, and I don't see why we shouldn't be able to rectify this situation. Since you have been officially removed from our provider list, Dr. Dackel, you will have to reapply, but I think it should go fairly smoothly if you send your application directly to me." There was another wink, this time directed at Dackel as he handed him a six page application. "Remember to send it to my attention and I'll do what I can to move it along."

They all shook hands and Dackel and Klee left.

"Smooth huh?" said Klee, all proud of himself.

"Did you see how fancy this place is?" said Dackel, "Did you see the art on the walls and that furniture. It pisses me off that they pay me shit and these guys have a facility like this. It just pisses me off!"

"Calm down dickhead, I got you back in didn't I?"

"I wish I could tell them to stick this application up their cost contained, mangled care asses," said Dackel. "These guys piss me off! Hey, thanks for coming."

"No problemo," shouted Klee as he got into his car.

Dackel called for his messages from the car. A patient had used Nair on her pubic area and was, as she put it, "as raw as chopped meat." Another wasn't sure if she had a urinary infection, a yeast infection, or whether she was allergic to new scented tampons that she had tried. A pre-certification reviewer called to say she was not approving a hysterectomy because there was inadequate documentation on the patient's chart. They were all typical calls. The last call, though, was from Carrie Bradford. He returned her call first.

"Hello?"

"Carrie?"

"Hi Dr. Dackel."

"How's everything going? Did you get the court order?"

"Not yet, there's been a snag."

"What kind of a snag?"

"The lawyer wants fifteen hundred dollars."

"Oh, Carrie, I hope you don't expect me to help you with that kind of money."

"I was hoping you would."

"It's out of the question. I couldn't possibly..."

"Dr. Dackel, I need the money."

"Carrie, I'm afraid I'm going to have to say no."

"I was hoping you would make this easy on yourself Dr. Dackel."

"I don't know what you mean."

"You will. Since you don't like the installment plan, perhaps you would prefer a lump sum payment," she said, her voice changing to the hard one she answered with the last time he called. "Check your mail in a few days." She hung up.

He sat there with the phone in his hand, driving almost without thinking where he was going. He pulled over to the side and hung up the phone.

"What the hell did I get myself into?" he said out loud. He wondered what he was going to get in the mail. What could she possibly have that would make her talk like that? He considered the possibility that her boyfriend was standing right there with a knife to her throat and that he made her say what she said. He figured that he would get a picture of him threatening her in the mail. He opened the door of his car and threw up in the gutter.

Dackel called Red in his car. “You gotta meet me at my office.”

“Can’t. Going out with Mildred. What’s up?”

“I don’t know, man, but I gotta talk to you tonight.”

“What do you mean you don’t know? What’s up?”

“I got a call from the girl I met in Florida and I think I’m into something deeper than I want to be.”

“I’ll call you as soon as I get home.”

As Dackel drove home he sensed the beginning of one of his headaches. They always started the same way, quietly and subtly—just a tiny area of tightness right below the bump behind his left ear. It was almost imperceptible and would sometimes stay that way for hours, but once he felt it, he knew there was nothing he could do about it regardless of how hard he rubbed it or what kind of pills he took. After a while it would spread across the back of his head and build slowly, very slowly, until he could feel it like a pulse. Then, over the next few hours the pulse would crescendo into a thumping and the thumping into a pounding and the pounding into a hammering. He would become nauseated and unfocused. He would have trouble concentrating. His skin would tingle. It would build until he got into bed and then the hammering would get so intense that he couldn’t bear it any more. He would take three or four Fiorinals, more than he knew he should take, more than he knew was a safe dose, and he’d finally fall asleep. The irony was that when he awoke the next morning he would feel rested, clear headed and generally terrific.

This was going to be one of those headaches. He was sure of it. He also had a subtle gnawing deep in his gut that was starting to build just like one of his headaches, but this was not a physical pain. It was more of a feeling that his world was about to turn completely to shit.

Dackel walked in the back door of his house and saw Arlene cooking dinner—real dinner. Veal marsala, his favorite—with real meat.

“What’s the occasion, hon?”

“Al, you’ve been so preoccupied lately, I just thought you might like a special treat.”

“That’s very nice of you,” he said, suddenly feeling guilty. He wasn’t sure where the guilt was coming from. He didn’t think it had anything to do with Carrie, the fact that he met her in a strip club, or the fact that he had coffee with her or that he even sent her money. He certainly wasn't romantically or even sexually interested in her— anymore.

The headache hadn't progressed enough to spoil his dinner, but shortly thereafter it shifted into overdrive. He apologized to Arlene and went up to bed. By nine it had hit the unbearable stage. He took two Fiorinals and laid another four out on his nightstand just in case he needed them. He fell asleep in twenty minutes.

At ten thirty the ringing of the phone hit him hard in the back of the head. The hammering returned with vengeance. The call was from Red.

"Okay crotchman, what's up?"

"I can't talk now, I'm in the middle of a stroke. I'll call you tomorrow."

"Some emergency," Red laughed as he hung up the phone. Yet he knew Dackel well enough to know that something important was up. He didn't know what was going to happen, but he knew it wasn't going to be good and he had a feeling that his buddy was about to be hurt.

Chapter 19

It was Thursday, operating day, but Dackel had no surgery scheduled. His cut in income was no longer hypothetical and he hoped his re-application to QHM would be processed quickly. On the other hand, it was rare that he had a day to himself. He normally would have called Red and gone to Atlantic City, but he knew Red was out of town on an audit.

He thought about his options. He could spend the day in the library and try to learn more about hysteroscopic endometrial ablation, but he learned better by watching. Besides, he would have MacDonald show him what to do when the time came. Besides, he had the literature from National. He could stay at home, but Arlene was hosting an artificial plant party that day. It was like a Tupperware party but they sold artificial plants instead. He thought for a second that it would be nice if she hosted a lingerie party, but then he figured it would be a waste. Even if she would wear sexy nightclothes to bed, her hair would probably still be full of clips and her face covered with goo.

He hated going to movies by himself so that was out, and he was finished with strip clubs for good. So he did something he had never done before. He took his beeper and his cellular phone and took a tour of the Liberty Bell, Betsy Ross' House, Independence Hall and four or five other Philadelphia Historical Landmarks. He had a wonderful time. It was interrupted at about one thirty by a patient in labor. He walked to the hospital and settled in for a long night. Fortunately for him, but unfortunately for her, the baby started to show signs of fetal distress and he had to perform a Caesarian Section. He was out of the hospital by six, with just enough time to grab dinner and get over to Deborah Metzger-Minkman's office.

The session was more of the same and he did very well.

"You're not going to need as much coaching as I thought," Deborah told him. "I even think we're ready to try a little radio interview. I'll pick a station that doesn't have a lot of listeners, and I'll get an early Sunday morning public affairs show.

I think I'll probably be able to set it up for next week. It won't really be the audience we want, but it will get you used to the studio, almost be like a dry run. It'll be fun, you'll see. I'll even come since it's the first time. No charge."

"What if they ask me something I don't know? Can I bring some books?" asked Dackel.

"Al, I know you're nervous, but you talk to patients every day. This is no different. You'll be fine."

He went home to a sleeping wife and a house full of new artificial plants.

Dackel was nervous about his first radio interview. He had gone through enough practice sessions with Deborah, but this was going to be live. She had arranged an interview at six AM on Sunday morning on WALT, an alternative rock station. The FCC requires that every radio station air some public affairs programming. Most stations schedule them for the least sellable time slot, which for this station was early Sunday morning. Metzger-Minkman thought this would be a good first experience mainly because she knew that no one would be listening. Nevertheless, Dackel was nervous. There would be no coach telling him "that was good, but say it another way."

The show was hosted by Kristie Knight, a cute 24 year-old kid, two years out of communications school. Her real name was Esther Michelle Meshansky, and until she would make her ultimate career move and accept a position co-anchoring the evening news for any one of the three major networks, she hosted a European alternative rock show from midnight to six. She was also responsible for opening the mail and sweeping the studio. She earned five dollars an hour with no benefits. Since she was there, she also had to do the Sunday public affairs show. They called this one "Philadelphia Alternatives," tying in the fact that WALT played alternative rock.

Metzger-Minkman pitched Dackel as an alternative gynecologist. Knight had expected a pony tailed young person in jeans who would talk about herbal cures for herpes and delivering babies under water. Instead she got Dackel, dressed in his dark blue suit with a powder blue shirt and a red, but not too busy, tie. He had dressed for television at Minkman's suggestion, "just to practice."

He arrived at the station at 5:30 in the morning and pressed the buzzer on the intercom for about ten minutes until a sleepy, scraggly kid in a very ripped tee shirt and very, very ripped jeans came to the door.

"Help you man?"

"Yes, I'm Dr. Alfred Dackel and I'm supposed to do a show at six."

"Yeah, that's twenty minutes from now, we didn't expect you so early. Come on in. Want some coffee or something?"

"No thank you, do you know if a Ms. Metzger-Minkman is here yet?"

"Debbie the flack? Nah, she's not here."

Deborah would explain to him later that a flack is the media's term for a publicist of any kind. The word came from an old tenacious bull dog of a record publicist whose last name was Flack or Flack-something.

"Wait here man, I mean Doc. Kristie will be with you in a few."

Dackel was ushered into a tiny room with posters all over the walls. He had never heard of any of the groups. The music playing in the background was also new to him. He waited nervously. At 5:55, still no Kristie and still no Metzger-Minkman, but just a minute later, they both walked in from opposite directions.

Minkman had in tow a sleepy eight year-old carrying a partially eaten bagel.

"Hi, my name's Kristie and I know your mommy, but what's your name?"

"Emma Beth Metzger-Minkman."

Dackel shook his head and sighed.

Deborah was wearing a pair of jeans and a "Save the Rain Forest" tee shirt. She must have been wearing a better bra because her breasts looked pretty good. If Red were there he would have said something very inappropriate like, "are you cold or just glad to see me?" or perhaps his other favorite line about headlights being on.

He was glad Red wasn't there because there is no telling what he would have said to Kristie Knight. She was 5'10", blond, and had an incredible body. She wore 40% of a tee shirt and had a ring in her belly button and a waist chain.

"Hi, are you the doctor?"

"Yes," he said, feeling even more nervous.

"Follow me, I have to read the news in about two minutes and then I'll introduce you." They walked toward the studio. "The demographics of this station are young. They're interested in birth control, sexually transmitted diseases and sex in general. I'll interview you for ten minutes and then we'll take calls—if anyone calls."

Dackel looked panicked. He glared at Metzger-Minkman. She smiled. She had a chive wedged between her two upper incisors and another one tooth over (to the left).

"This isn't what we talked about. She doesn't want to hear about endometrial ablation," Dackel whispered to Deborah.

"It's good practice Al," she whispered back, getting pleasantly close to Dackel's ear, "it will prepare you for the real interviews. Listen this isn't brain surgery, the worst you can do is say something stupid, but you won't. I trained you well. You'll be fine." Besides, nobody's listening, she said to herself.

Dackel and Kristie went into the studio and Deborah and Emma Beth Metzger-Minkman went back to the tiny room.

"Stand by," said a voice from behind the glass belonging to the guy who let Dackel into the building.

Kristie started her news. Dackel didn't really pay attention. He was nervous and pissed off. He wasn't prepared to talk about anything other than ablation. Kristi got his attention and motioned for him to put on his headphones.

"In other news, the construction on I-95 continues, closing one lane in each direction. PennDot spokesperson, Matthew Kelly, says that we can expect to see both lanes re-open sometime next month. Here's a statement from Matthew Kelly from a news conference held on Friday."

[Kelly's voice] "We can expect to see both lanes re-open sometime next month."

"And that's all the news from The Alternative, WALT in Philadelphia. It's time now for 'Philadelphia Alternatives', a public affairs program brought to you by WALT." [music: Purcell's Trumpet Voluntary, standard public affairs music]

"My guest today on "Philadelphia Alternatives" is alternative gynecologist, Dr. Albert Darden from the Fourteenth Street Hospital. Good morning, Dr. Darden."

"It's Dackel, Dr. Alfred Dackel," he said hesitantly. Metzger-Minkman had taught him what to do if a host mispronounced his name. Neither of them expected that she would be so far off, but he handled it fairly well. Actually, she had told him to make the correction quickly and go directly on to something else. That way it saves the host from having to make a big deal out of apologizing. He would have gone on, but he just didn't know where to go.

"I'm sorry, Dr. Dackel, I know it's early for you, but I've been up all night." Obviously, no one had ever coached Ms. Knight on how to handle a mispronounced name. She should have said a quick, "I'm sorry," and moved on.

She took a Magic Marker and wrote **DACKEL** in large black letters on a coffee stained napkin. "Dr. Dackel, one of the issues confronting young women today is genital warts. Can you tell us a little about what causes them, how you treat them and what to do to prevent them?"

"Where did this kid go to communications school?" Deborah rhetorically asked her eight-year-old daughter. Even you know better than that, don't you?"

"Yes mommy," replied Emma. "She should ask one question at a time so that she stays in control."

"Right!" she said, leaning over and giving her a kiss on the head.

Dackel decided to try his newly learned techniques. "Genital warts is an important issue, but there is an even more important one that I think needs to be discussed first, Kristie."

"And what is that, Dr. Dar-Dackel?"

She went for the hook. Dave Evans was right and Deborah's credibility was re-established. "I think there are too many hysterectomies being performed today."

Knight then used a bridge of her own. "Yes, I guess that's important for some audiences, but our audience is too young for hysterectomies, so lets talk about genital warts."

"So much for media training," he thought. Metzger-Minkman was listening from the tiny room. She screwed up and she knew it. She just hoped that he could pull it off.

"Genital warts," said Dackel, are caused by a virus called the HPV or human papilloma virus. They're sexually transmitted and highly contagious." He went on to describe the symptoms, treatments and after effects of the infection, and he did a very good job.

After a few questions from Kristie, they took a few phone calls and then the show was over. She thanked Dackel, asked if she could switch to him as her gynecologist because the one she was going to could not get rid of her warts, and invited him to come back in a month to talk about herpes.

Metzger-Minkman prepared for the worst. "Emma honey," she whispered, "when Dr. Dackel comes in here he may be upset, and he may even yell at mommy. Don't let it upset you."

But that never happened. Dackel walked into the tiny room with a smile on his face. "Hello ladies," he said, "did you enjoy the show? I thought it was pretty good. May I buy you two breakfast at The International House of Pancakes?"

Metzger-Minkman was shocked. "You're not upset?" she asked.

"Why should I be?" he answered. "I think I got a lot of good information out, and how about those callers? I really think I helped that last one." There was more enthusiasm in Dackel's voice than Deborah had ever heard.

"I just thought that since she didn't let you talk about the ablation, that you might be upset..."

"Upset, I was actually relieved. I got to talk about something I really know about, Deborah, and it felt good. To be honest, I'm not really sure about this ablation thing. I think I need more experience before I pretend to be an expert."

"Well you better get it by next week because 'Morning in Philly' is going to interview you on Friday."

They went to breakfast at IHOP. He loved their coffee. Emma had pancakes that Deborah decorated like a clown face using butter and syrup. To anyone watching, they looked like a very happy family.

Chapter 20

On Monday morning the Shintocks were back to talk about Linda's bleeding.

"Linda, I've gone over your records and I see that your doctor has done everything she could think of to try to regulate your bleeding. As I see it, you have one of three alternatives. You can let it be, take iron to keep your blood count up and hope that it fixes itself. Another option would be a hysterectomy. In your case, I could do it through the vagina. It would take me about forty minutes and you'd be out of the hospital in a day or two. Or, you could consider endometrial ablation, the new operation that we discussed last time you were here. I have some additional information for you and you can take a look at a video tape that shows how it's done."

He played the tape for Linda and Paul while he stepped out of the room to see another patient. When he returned, they told him that they had made a decision. They wanted the ablation with the DAC-III.

"I like the idea that I can keep my uterus and that I'll only be in the hospital for a few hours. Besides, it looks like it's a safer operation," Linda said with more confidence than Dackel had.

"Yes, statistically it is safer," Dackel said, "but there are still risks. You could get an infection, there could be an injury to the uterus, it might not even work. But yes, it looks like it is safer and it will definitely be easier on you than a hysterectomy. Your other doctor has already given you Depo-Lupron to shrink the uterine lining so if we do the procedure within a week or two, you won't need another shot."

"Thank goodness," said Linda. "These hot flashes from the Lupron are killer. The sooner the better."

"If you have any questions or you change your mind, call me," said Dackel, half-wishing she would change her mind. His excitement about learning a new procedure was being overtaken by his fear of doing a new procedure with which he was not yet comfortable.

While his secretary called the scheduling office to set up the admission for that Thursday, Dackel called National and asked for MacDonald.

"Mark? Al Dackel from Philadelphia. I set up one of those ablations. She fits all the criteria for the study and she's hot for it. It's scheduled for Thursday. I understand you're going to come up for the first one just to make sure everything's set up right."

"I'll be there. I have to be up north next week anyway. I'll come in on Wednesday night and fly out Thursday after the procedure. Can you get a 7:30 start?"

"Sure can, it's my priority day," said Dackel proudly. Only the senior attendings got guaranteed early O.R. starts.

Later that day, Deborah Metzger-Minkman called to give Dackel the details for Friday and he told her he felt better about the interview because he would be doing his first case on Thursday.

"I have a great idea," she said, "I'll call you back." She hung up. Ten minutes later she was back on the phone.

"Wait till you hear this, Al, they're going to send a crew to film your first case on Thursday. It will be great. If she agrees, they'll interview your patient before and after, and they'll be taking pictures, discretely, of course, while you're doing the operation. Then, the next day you'll go to the studio and talk about it, and if your patient is up to it, she'll be on too. It will be wonderful publicity."

"I don't know, Deborah, my first case, I'm not sure..."

"Listen Al, these people are friends of mine. It's what we call a 'warm fuzzy' show. They're not out to get you. I told them you would absolutely have to approve any video b-roll that goes on the air.

"What's b-roll?" Dackel asked impatiently.

"Oh, I'm sorry," Deborah said, "it's a television term from the old days. When they're interviewing you, the film of you and the interviewer would be called the a-roll, like roll of film. Any film that they cut in during the course of the interview, would be called b-roll."

"Well, I'm trusting you on this one, but I still think I'd rather wait till I have a couple of these under my belt before..."

"Al, if you trust me, then trust me."

"I trust you." He did.

The week went quickly and it was Wednesday before he knew it. As it got later in the day, he began to feel anxious. He was starting to experience almost the same feelings that he had lied to Capuston about. He didn't sleep well Wednesday night. It happened occasionally the night before a case that he anticipated would be difficult. He would go to bed at the usual time, eleven or eleven thirty. He would usually fall asleep right away, but then in an hour or so he would suddenly awaken from a dream which was always about something that was going wrong during the case. It was often something silly like his mask would keep falling off or the nurse would keep handing him the wrong instruments. Those were frustrating dreams. The scary ones were the ones where the patient was bleeding and he couldn't stop it or her blood pressure kept dropping and they couldn't figure out why.

He had these dreams when he was younger. When he was a child, it would usually be one of two scenarios, either someone was chasing him and he was trying to get into his house but he couldn't find the right key, or he was trying to call the police and he kept dialing the wrong number.

After he got into college his worst dream was that it was finals week and he had forgotten to go to a class the whole semester. Now that he was a doctor, it was either the bleeding, or the dropping blood pressure dreams that woke him in cold sweats and with palpitations. This particular night it was a new one. He dreamed that he couldn't see anything through the hysteroscope and he didn't remember how to work the DAC-III.

Once he was awakened by one of these dreams, he knew that was it for the night. He would fall asleep again, but the same dream would wake him over and over. It was worse than staying up all night with a labor patient. At least you had something to do and someone to talk to. With these dreams, you're never really awake, and never really asleep. You really are stuck in a twilight zone where the same bad thing keeps happening, and happening and happening.

The interesting thing is that when they perform sleep lab tests on people who have this kind of insomnia, they often find that they do sleep quite a lot between awakenings and yet they perceive that that they hadn't slept at all. Dackle thought he had been up all night, yet when the alarm rang at 5:30, he was definitely sound asleep.

He got out of bed exhausted. His eyes hurt and it was painful to open them. He shuffled to the bathroom. It looked brighter than usual even though he hadn't yet turned on the light.

"Oh no," he thought, "I hope it isn't..." he parted the curtains and looked out the bathroom window. It was. The glare made his eyes hurt more. The glare was from at least a foot of snow that had fallen overnight. But it looked as if it had stopped and his street was already plowed. He could also count on his Bronco to get him to the hospital. He would swing by the Marriott and pick up MacDonald who had been scheduled to arrive late Wednesday night.

He dressed, kissed Arlene and stopped in the kitchen to prepare his breakfast which he ate on the way. A bagel with fat free cream cheese (the only kind available in the Dackel house), and an apple or preferably a banana. Dackel actually liked apples better but the juicy ones would sometimes drip on his shirt. Bananas were neater. He downed a large glass of orange juice and took the rest to his truck. Luckily, it started. It didn't always. Once he pulled out of the driveway, he turned on Howard Stern, opened his glove compartment and took out a pack of sugar and cinnamon Pop Tarts just in case he was still hungry after the bagel and the banana. He couldn't remember the last time that he wasn't.

He drove to the Marriott, parked on the side of the circular driveway and went into the lobby where MacDonald was supposed to have been waiting. Dackel didn't see him. He picked up a house phone and asked for his room. The operator told him that she had no one registered by that name. Panicking, he walked over to the front desk, and asked whether a Dr. MacDonald had checked in. He hadn't but according to their records, he would be arriving today, and yes, there was a message for a Dr. Bracken.

"That must be me," he said asking for the message.

It read, "Sorry I got delayed in Providence. Will meet you in the hospital by nine."

"Nine, the surgery is scheduled for seven thirty," he said to the desk clerk who shrugged his shoulders.

Dackel got in the truck and called the O.R. on his cellular. He told the charge nurse that his case would be delayed about an hour and a half.

"That's okay, I anticipate that some of the staff will be late anyway," she said. "This is the case you need that new machine for, right?"

"Jesus Christ Meg, I called yesterday to make sure it was there and ready for me."

"Hold your pants on, Al, it's ready, I was just making sure. A nurse from National was down last week training Margie on how to set it up."

Long gone were the days that nurses respected doctors just because they were doctors. Besides, Meg Finney had been around 14th Street as long as Dackel and they were actually pretty good friends.

"Al, isn't this the case that the guy from Florida is coming in for?"

"Yeah, he's probably landing right now," said Dackel.

"Not in our airport he's not," laughed Meg.

"What do you mean?"

"I mean if you would listen to a normal station instead of that idiot you're always talking about, you would have heard that the airport is closed."

Dackel suddenly felt an urgent need for a bathroom. He hung up without a good-bye, ran back into the hotel and, in a marble bathroom just off the lobby, he emptied his intestines from the neck down in one explosive wave. He would have to cancel the case. His patient and the press would have to understand. His beeper went off. He called his service and was patched into MacDonald, calling from Rhode Island.

"Dr. Dackel, I'm sorry, I had a 6:30 flight, but the airport is closed. I can't get out. You're going to have to do it without me, but you'll be fine."

"I won't be fine, I'm going to cancel the case," Dackel screamed. "I don't know the equipment or the procedure well enough."

"Al, please don't cancel. We're counting on you to get this on the news tonight. We have a stockholders meeting tomorrow and it would look great if we could show them that the machine is out there and functioning. It's easy. All you have to do is put the scope in. Your nurses have been trained to do the rest. Trust me, it's easy. I'll also stick by the phone and I'll talk you through it. Just tell the news people that they can photograph the unit and the O.R. but they can't record any sound during the case. You can put me on speaker and it'll be just like having me there. It's a shame we didn't have enough notice to set up a virtual surgery link. Then I could actually watch or help if I had to, but, you know, if you can get somebody with a digital camera, you can shoot me images over the Internet. Call your computer systems guys, maybe they can set it up."

"I don't know, Mark, I just don't know."

He hung up and headed for the hospital. He thought of calling someone for advice, but who? Red didn't understand this stuff. He would say, "hey you took the course, go do it." Arlene would say a lot but not offer any usable advice. Capuston would just sit there and shake his vegetarian head. Deborah was the only one who he thought could help, but it was too early for her to be in her office and he had neither her phone number nor the guts to dial it even if he did.

He got to the hospital without any problem and went directly up to the O.R. holding area to talk to his patient. The crew from Morning in Philly were already interviewing Linda Shintock. Dackel asked them for some privacy.

"Linda, we may be having some trouble with the DAC-III equipment today, and there's a chance we might have to cancel your surgery."

"Oh, Dr. Dackel, no. I took off tomorrow and Monday and I can't change that, my mother flew in from Phoenix to take care of the kids, and remember I told you my company is switching my insurance to QHM in four days and you're not on their list. Can't you use one of the other methods of ablation that they talked about when I saw you on the tape?"

"Let me see what I can do," he said, heading for the bathroom again with an urgency that made him think that Montezuma himself was chasing him. The other methods were out of the question. He had never even seen them performed. This one he had at least done, albeit on a life-sized Barbie Doll. It wasn't really that hard, and MacDonald did say he'd stand by on the phone.

He decided to go for it. He paged the administrator on call and told her to do what she had to do to get a digital video camera and hook it up to the hospital's Internet server. She told him that the computer guys made it in, but the videographer didn't. He told her he'd call her back. He went back to the holding area and had a brief conversation with the TV crew. Then he went over to talk with his patient.

"I have to be honest with you Linda, I haven't used this particular machine before except in a training setting and the medical director from the company was going to come down and make sure everything was set up properly, but he got snowed in. The TV crew is trying to link up to him by Internet and he's going to check us out that way."

"There's not going to be a cameraman in the room is there?" Linda asked.

"No, Linda, he's just going to set up the camera on a tripod and leave the room."

"Oh, then that's fine. Dr. Dackel, I trust you. I saw you on the tape and I heard that you were even on the radio, and I know you're a good doctor. Why else would they have named the machine after you?"

"They—they didn't really name it after...would you like to discuss this with your husband? Perhaps he..."

"No, this is my decision and I really appreciate it that you're going to go ahead today. I feel safe in your hands."

She smiled as she took one of those hands she felt safe in and squeezed it. He still remembers the words, the smile and the squeeze. They are his new nightmare.

By 9:30 the digital video camera was set up on a tripod in the corner of the operating room and hooked up through an Ethernet connection to the hospital's mainframe. A connection had been established to National's headquarters in Tampa and routed to MacDonald's Powerbook, which he had set up in an airport motel in Providence.

"Where's Meg?" Dackel asked.

"She's snowbound, Dr. Dackel," replied Anna Nichols. "She lives all the way out in New Hope and she called to say that even with her 4 wheel she couldn't make it out of her driveway. I usually work in ENT, but all their cases canceled so they sent me over. But don't worry, Meg filled me in on the machine. It's pretty easy. There's nothing much to know. Just tell me what solution you want for irrigation."

"What are my choices?"

"The usual," she said, walking over to the shelf piled high with various bags of fluid. You can use physiologic saline, dextrose and water, glycine, sorbitol, mannitol, let's see what else is up here. How about this one, it says "Sterile Water for Irrigation."

Dackel thought about it for a minute. He remembered that the magnetic resonance spectroscopy part of the procedure had something to do with recognizing different chemicals and all of the solutions had chemicals in them except for the "Sterile Water for Irrigation." Yes, that made the most sense to him.

"Let's try these," he said, pulling out two bags of water. Do you know how to hook it up?"

"Sure, the instructions are right on the machine. You just push these spikes into the bottom of the bags like this, and, see, it's done. Why don't you go scrub."

"Fine. Where's my resident?"

"Oh, I forgot to tell you, Dr. Washington called. She said they're really short today because of the snow and there are preemie breech twins in labor so they're sending down a first year to help you."

"Unacceptable!" he yelled, "I need a senior resident for this case. A first year is unacceptable. Call her back right now."

Dackel was counting on a senior resident to help him with the hysteroscopic part of the procedure. His residents had grown up with hysteroscopy and they all seemed very comfortable with it. He was hoping to have the resident do the hysteroscopy while he acted like he was teaching her how to do it. He hadn't counted on a first year. A first year would be no help.

"I'm sorry, Dr. Dackel," said Anna returning after a few minutes, "I just called up there and they said Washington just started a C-section and she has two more patients that are probably going to deliver within the hour, but Dr. Dimucci is on his way."

"Who's that? Is he a first year? I never heard of Dimucci."

"I wouldn't know," said Anna, "I usually work in ENT."

As they wheeled Linda Shintock into OR room 7, she was already feeling the first effects of the midazolam, a Valium type medicine that has become a popular pre-op drug because of its ability to cause temporary amnesia. Patients are sedated and even groggy but they are awake and cooperative. They can move from the gurney to the operating table. They can ask and answer questions but after the operation they don't remember a damn thing. As she passed by the scrub sink where Dackel was washing his hands, she gave him a half of a smile and a quarter of a wave.

Arnie Geller was the anesthesiologist. He knew that Dackel was a bit old fashioned and not up on all the latest techniques, but he respected him as a surgeon. He had introduced himself to Linda in the holding area where he took her history, listened to her heart and lungs and started her intravenous. He concluded that she was a class 1A patient at very low risk for anesthesia complications. Geller usually was assigned to the more complicated patients but the snow had caused all kinds of schedule and personnel changes.

The holding area nurse had already started her IV. Geller put some sticky electrodes on her chest and the sides of her abdomen and clipped wires to them, which hooked her up to an EKG machine, to monitor her heart rate and rhythm during the case. He clipped a device onto the end of her index finger that looked like a plastic clothespin. This was a pulse oxymeter, which also measures heart rate but, more importantly, instantaneously estimates the amount of oxygen in the blood. It works by shining a red light through the skin and measuring the reflection of that light. At any particular time, an individual blood cell may or may not be carrying oxygen. The percentage of blood cells that contain oxygen is called the oxygen saturation level. For a healthy person, it is usually 99% or greater. If the body begins to have problems getting oxygen, it attempts to prioritize oxygen delivery. The blood supply to the fingers is one of the first things it shuts down. Fortunately, the brain is one of the last. The important thing is that knowing the oxygen saturation level in the finger can be an early warning sign of trouble.

In the days before the pulse ox, you had to draw blood from an artery (not a vein), keep it on ice and run it immediately to the lab in order to get that information.

"Linda, I'm going to put a mask on your face and give you some oxygen to breathe." The idea was to fill the lungs and saturate the blood with oxygen before the patient went to sleep. Once she did, he would then inject another drug that would paralyze her and stop her breathing. He would then put a tube into her trachea or wind pipe and hook it up to a pump that would breathe for her. Pre-oxygenating her assured that she would have enough oxygen going to her brain during the short time between when she stopped breathing on her own and when the respirator took over. It also allowed Arnie more time to get the tube in.

After a few minutes he took a syringe of a milky white solution called propofol, hooked it up to a stopcock that he had inserted in the IV line and started to inject.

"This is going to burn a little, Linda."

It did. She grimaced, and then she was out.

"Linda, can you take a deep breath?"

She couldn't. That was one of the ways he could tell she was asleep. He then ran his index finger lightly across her eyelashes. She didn't move. That was trick number two. He injected another syringe of medicine, the one that would paralyze her. It only took a few seconds. As her breathing became shallow, he squeezed a rubber bag forcing air into her lungs. As the paralyzing drug took full effect, he could feel that the bag became easier to squeeze. That meant that her muscles were paralyzed and could not resist the flow of oxygen that was being forced into her lungs.

He took a quick look at the monitors and picked up his laryngoscope, basically a flashlight with a blunt metal blade on the top to push the tongue out of the way. He tilted her head back and put the scope in her mouth and pulled up on her bottom jaw, temporarily and purposefully dislocating it. He looked into her throat and visualized her vocal folds, which used to be called vocal cords. They looked like two rubber bands. Without taking his eyes off the folds, he reached over and picked up the endotracheal tube, which was just where he always left it. He expertly slipped the tube down her throat right between the folds, and then he injected air through a small plastic valve, which blew up a small balloon called a cuff, that kept air from leaking around the tube. He hooked the tube to an automatic respirator, which would pump just the right amount of oxygen, nitrous oxide and other anesthetic gasses into the lungs at just the right pressure and with just the right frequency. He let out an unconscious sigh. Once the tube is positioned and taped, barring complications, an anesthesiologist can usually relax until his next important job, waking the patient up and taking out the tube.

Geller was a pilot. He considered the anesthesia induction like a take off and the waking up like a landing. He was a good pilot and a good anesthesiologist.

"Okay, you can put her up now." Arnie said as Dackel walked into the room. "Hey Al, you're branching out. I didn't know you did ablations."

"You gotta move with the times, Arnie."

Anna took Linda's legs, one at a time and placed them in the stirrups, exposing her vulva to the immediate world, which couldn't have cared less. She had shaved herself according to Dackel's instructions.

The telephone rang.

"Put it on speaker, its probably MacDonald," ordered Dackel. "Hello?"

"Dr. Dackel, it's Mark MacDonald. Can you hear me?"

"Yes, I can hear you fine. Is the video working?"

"Yep, we've had it up for about a half-hour. Your people did a great job. I can see you and your patient on half the screen and on the other half they're going to send me a feed from the hysteroscope camera. Your crew is pretty impressive." Apparently MacDonald didn't know that the television crew did all the hooking up and feeding and whatever else they had to do. "What we did is we had them send the signal to Donny Moline in our Tampa studio. He's fooling with it and sending it up to me. Isn't the net amazing?"

"Yeah. We're going to get started."

"Before you do, do you have any questions about setting up the machine?"

"No Dr. MacDonald," replied Anna, "it's pretty straight forward."

The scrub nurse, Dan Alverez, an ex Navy corpsman, held out Dackel's gown while Dackel slipped his arms through the sleeves. Anna tied the gown in the back. Dan then gloved him.

"Where the hell is my resident? he yelled as Sal Dimucci walked in the door.

"I'm sorry, Dr. Dackel, things are crazy upstairs. I came as soon as I could," said Dimucci with a pea soup thick Brooklyn accent.

"Go out and scrub. You're not any help to me just standing there with your teeth in your mouth," scowled Dackel. Dimucci left to scrub for six minutes and by the time he returned, Dackel had prepped the patient with a generic brand of Betadine, an iodine solution. Then he draped her with paper drapes, first one leg, then the other. He was nervous.

Dimucci came into the room, gowned and gloved and stood by Dackel's side.

"Have you seen an endometrial ablation yet son?"

"No sir, this is my first."

"Well, I'll tell you what I'm doing step by step."

Dackel's real reason for doing that was so MacDonald could hear what he was about to do before he did it. Hopefully this would keep him out of trouble.

"The first step in any gynecologic surgery is to do a bimanual examination. I'm going to put two fingers into her vagina and my other hand above her pubic bone and I'm going to palpate or feel the organs between them. I should be able to feel the uterus and, in a patient who's not too fat or too old, I should be able to feel the ovaries."

"I understand too fat, but why can't you feel them in an older person?"

"It's February Dimucci, has your head been up your ass for seven months?"

"No sir, I just started mid year. I broke my back right after graduation and I was in bed for a couple months."

"Oh, sorry to hear. The reason you can't feel ovaries in an old lady is that they shrink. Now you examine her."

Dimucci tentatively inserted the first two fingers of his right hand deep into Linda's vagina and pushed on her abdomen, rather delicately with his left hand.

"What do you feel, son?"

"I-I'm not sure."

"Can you feel the uterus?"

"I can't be sure."

"Can you feel anything?"

"Well..."

"Dimucci, can you feel that one hand is warmer than the other?"

Dimucci looked quizzically at Dackel and then started to smile. Then Dackel and the rest of the room started to laugh. There were also chuckles coming from the speakerphone.

"You'll get it soon. Step aside. Now I'm putting in the speculum to hold the vagina open, and I'm going to grab the top lip of the cervix, see the cervix, with this tenaculum."

MacDonald was listening intently. He heard the clang of the metal speculum and then the ratchet of the tenaculum as he watched on his laptop. The way the camera was angled, he couldn't see much but he wasn't at all worried about this part of the procedure. It was standard for many types of gyn surgery.

"Now I'm going to sound the uterus. That means I'm going to put this metal probe in as far as it can go. The sound has a ruler on it so I'll be able to measure the depth of the uterine cavity. Here we go, eight centimeters. Now I'm going to dilate. How much Mark?" he said raising his voice and turning his head towards the telephone.

"The scope is 10 millimeters, you need to go to 31 French, but don't overdilate or you'll get a leak. French was a measuring system that was used with many medical devices. Each millimeter equaled three French units.

"Thanks. Dimucci, see these dilators? They're all marked. You start with the real thin ones, and you keep using bigger and bigger ones 'till you get to the dilation that you need. Hand me the next one."

"Okay Mark, she's dilated to 31."

"Now take the scope Al. It's already hooked to the camera. Start the flow of the fluid Anna, that's the first button. It says flow."

Fluid started running out the end of the scope.

"Anna, turn on the light. That's the next button, and Al, insert the scope through the cervix. Look at the monitor. You'll see a red area. That's where the lens is up against tissue. When you see that, don't push any more or you'll perf. Aim for the black. That's the canal. I can see what you're doing, go ahead."

There was silence for a few moments and then MacDonald spoke again. "Al, aim up a little. You see the black on the top of the monitor? That's the canal. Go easy. Aim up a little more."

"Dimucci, can you see? asked Dackel.

"Not really sir," he answered.

"Well then move to a spot where you can see."

Dimucci started to move to other side but on the way, he tripped on a TV cable and fell against the DAC-III. Dackel's screen suddenly went black.

"Shit, what's going on here? I lost my picture!" yelled Dackel.

MacDonald cut in, "Al, I still have a picture, it must be your monitor. Check your monitor. Meanwhile, take the camera off of the scope and look directly through the eyepiece."

"Will somebody fix the television," he said unclipping the camera from the scope.

"MacDonald spoke. Okay, Al, I can't see now because the camera's off. When you get your TV working put the camera back on. In the meantime, take a look around the uterus and see what's going on, and don't push any buttons."

There was mass confusion in the room. Anna was trying to figure what went wrong with the television. Dackel was holding an instrument he had held only once before, and doing an operation he had never done on a real patient. Dimucci was untangling himself from a web of wires. MacDonald saw and heard the commotion and took charge.

"Okay everyone, settle down. No need to panic. Anna, check the wire from the camera control box to the monitor and check the monitor power cord. Al, what do you see."

"I see blood."

"Do you see blood or do you see red tissue?"

"It's blood, and there's some leaking out around the scope."

"Hook the camera back up so I can see what's going on. Anna, how're we coming?

"There are so many wires."

"Anna," said MacDonald calmly, "go to the television monitor. Is the power light on?"

"Where's the power light?"

"Do you see any lights?"

"No."

"Okay Anna, go to the back of the television. There should be two cords. One plugs into the VCR and the other one plugs into the power strip. Follow the cords and see if they're plugged in. Al I got a picture. I know you can't see but hopefully Anna will have us up in a minute. There is a lot of blood, turn up the pressure of the irrigating fluid to try to flush it out."

Anna found the power cord and plugged it back in. The television flickered and then came on. All anyone saw was red. There was also a small puddle collecting by Dackel's feet.

"The irrigation's turned all the way up, Mark, I can't see anything."

"Neither can I."

That's when her blood pressure started to drop. Geller asked what was going on. Dackel didn't know. MacDonald was no help. Geller tried turning up her IV and injecting ephedrine to try to maintain her blood pressure. It didn't work.

"We're losing her Al. Take out the scope and see how much she's bleeding."

He removed the hysteroscope. There was a gush of blood but it lasted for only a few seconds. Then it seemed to stop.

"It's letting up Arnie, I think we're okay."

"We're not okay Al, she's not bleeding because her heart stopped. Call a code, get me six units of universal blood stat and get her feet down. Al, if you think you perfed, get ready to open her."

Arnie pulled off the drapes and started pumping her chest. In moments, the room was filled. Two more anesthesiologists, a cardiologist and the nursing supervisor all came in and started doing what they had done all too many times. Each had his or her job. The team functioned smoothly and efficiently, but, this time, not successfully. They worked on Linda for twenty minutes with no response.

"I can't understand it," Arnie said. She was bleeding, but not enough to kill her, and we were on top of things. I can't figure out why we lost her. First her pressure went up, then the bottom dropped out."

At the other end of the Internet connection, MacDonald was frozen. He didn't know exactly what had happened, but he was pretty sure that it wouldn't have happened if he had been there. Donny Moline watched the whole thing from his control room. When the shit started heading for the fan, he called up to the executive offices to alert them. About six of National's top executives jammed into the control room to follow the disaster as it was happening. No one thought about the television crew.

Geller and Dackel walked to the surgical family waiting room. There were six or seven families, each waiting for a call telling them that their loved one's operation was over and everything was all right. It's generally a tense but ultimately happy place, with one family after another breathing collective sighs of relief after talking to the surgeons. Today would be different.

They approached Paul Shintock. He got out of his chair and walked to them smiling. When they didn't return the smile he suspected something was wrong. He guessed that they had to do a hysterectomy.

Dackel had learned over the years that the best way to do what he had to do was to say it directly. Euphemisms like "didn't make it" or "passed" were sometimes misunderstood.

"Paul, there were some complications and I'm sorry to say that Linda died."

They waited. They knew what would be next. They were right. First there was silence for what seemed like minutes but was probably seconds. Then there was denial.

"That's impossible. Are you sure? There must be some mistake."

Elisabeth Kubler-Ross wrote the classic treatise on death and dying. In it she explains that people go through universal stages when they lose a loved one. The first stage is denial.

Geller spoke, "Mr. Shintock, I'm Dr. Geller from anesthesia. We're not really sure yet what happened, but I can tell you that we did all we could, and that she died without any pain."

You would think that a statement like that was self serving and even trite, but you would be amazed how many times in the next few weeks Paul Shintock repeated those words as comfort to himself and to those who offered condolences.

Dackel went back to the operating suite. By the time he got there, there was another case going on in OR 7. He went into the locker room and changed into his street clothes. He sat down at a desk, dialed a number and spoke to a machine at a machine gun pace. He had dictated so many operative notes over the years that the first part of the dictation spilled out automatically, sounding like one run-on sentence.

"This is Dr. Alfred Dackel dictating an operative report on Linda Shintock, S-h-i-n-t-o-c-k, medical record 856675. Date of surgery was February 19th. Preoperative diagnosis was intractable uterine bleeding. Post operative diagnosis was same. Indication for surgery was heavy menstrual bleeding not controlled by hormonal manipulation or D&C. Surgeon was Dr. Alfred Dackel, assistant was Dr. Sal Dimucci, anesthesia was general. Intravenous fluid was 2000 cc. plasmalyte, estimated blood loss was 750 cc. Procedure: Hysteroscopy and attempted endometrial ablation. The patient was placed on the operating table and after satisfactory induction of general endotracheal anesthesia she was placed in the dorsal lithotomy position prepped and draped in the usual manner. Bimanual examination was performed revealing a top normal size uterus and normal adnexae. A weighted speculum was placed in the vagina. The anterior lip of the cervix was grasped with a single toothed tenaculum and the uterus was sounded to eight centimeters. The cervix was then dilated to 31 French to accept a DAC-III hysteroscope. The hysteroscope was inserted without difficulty and visualization was adequate."

His pace suddenly slowed up. His speech halting. "The—uh monitor suddenly-uh—mal-malfunctioned so the—the—uh uterine cavity was examined through the eyepiece of the telescope. At—uh— that time there was a-uh-small—no make that a mod-moderate amount of bleeding noted from the —uh cervix. The pressure on the hysteroscope pump was turned up in an attempt to flush the blood."

By now he was mumbling and speaking in almost a whisper. "At this point a cardiac arrest occurred and the instruments were removed. Attempts at resuscitation were futile and at 9:50 AM on 2/19/96 the patient was pronounced deceased by Arnold Geller, M.D. and myself. End of dictation on Linda Shintock. This is Dr. Alfred Dackel."

Chapter 21

By this time the streets were plowed. Dackel got into his truck and started to drive. He called Red because he had to talk to someone.

"I'm afraid of what the autopsy might show," he said, "I don't even know what I did, but I'm sure it was my fault. I never should have let them talk me into doing the case today."

"Can't you do something about the autopsy?" asked Red.

"What are you talking about?"

"You know."

"No I don't know. What do you mean do something. An autopsy is an autopsy, and this one is a medical examiner's case." yelled Dackel, loud enough to make the driver of the mail truck that was stopped next to him look over.

"What the hell's a medical examiner's case?" Red asked.

"Any suspicious death or any surgical death is a is a medical examiner's case. That means that an autopsy must be done, and the M.E. himself can demand to do it. Usually they let the hospital pathologist do it, but not always."

"Well you know the pathologists, can't they help you pull a 'Pretty Boy'?" asked Red.

Dackel thought for a moment and then it clicked. Red was referring to an incident that happened forty-five years ago.

"You're out of your mind! That's not an answer and I could go to jail if I got caught, you stupid bastard. You're a lot of fucking help!" He let out a one-syllable snort of disbelief. "I'll talk to you later, crazy man," he said shaking his head, still not sure whether Red was serious or not.

He hung up the phone, disgusted at how Red thought more about the consequences than the death. But then he actually cracked a smile for the first time that day, and the last time that month. Pretty Boy, he thought. Although he hadn't thought about Pretty Boy for years, he remembered it as clearly as any memory he had. He even remembered the date, forty-five years ago, February 15th, the day after Valentine's Day. Al and Red were thirteen years old and both had a crush on Carolyn Primmet. She was also thirteen, but there were parts of her that were matured well beyond her years. She had been one of the first in the class to develop making her the boy's first contemporary with any degree of significant breastage. They didn't call it that back then. As best as he could recall, they called them knockers or knobs.

Dackel got sidetracked for a moment thinking about the power of breasts, and the effects they had on him and his buddy, and probably every other man alive, be he thirteen or fifty eight. He wondered if girls had a similar universal preoccupation.

Pretty Boy. It was the day after Valentine's day and Carolyn, who lived on their street, had invited them in to play a game. She liked to play games, especially Chinese Checkers and Sorry!. He didn't remember which they were going to play that night. He thought it may have been Sorry!, but it didn't matter because they never got to play anything.

Red knocked on the door and then just pushed it open as was the custom in the neighborhood. No one ever locked the door back then. There was no need to. Unfortunately, Pretty Boy who was Caroline's blue and green parakeet, and, because of her allergies her only pet, was out of his cage at that moment enjoying a brief sortie around the living room. Now, you would think that a tropical bird that was smart enough to say seven different words, imitate the sound of a telephone ringing and recreate a very realistic burp and a truly convincing fart (compliments of Carolyn's brother) would be smart enough not to fly out into two degree weather. But if you thought that, you would be wrong. Pretty Boy flew out the door and headed north. Apparently, he couldn't get anything right.

Carolyn was frantic. She insisted that the boys help her try to find him. She put on her coat and boots and the three of them walked around the neighborhood until they couldn't feel their toes anymore. The search was called off after about an hour. Carolyn was a bright kid and mentally as well as physically mature. Back in her kitchen, between gulps of hot chocolate and bursts of tears, she faced the probability that Pretty Boy would not make it through the night. The boys agreed and pledged that they would get up at dawn the next day and find him so they could at least honor him with a proper burial. They were not inexperienced with pet funerals.

The following day they were up at the crack of nine and they scoured the area thoroughly for the remains of the bird. At about nine twenty, after an exhaustive search, Red came up with one of his most brilliant plans ever. They ran to the pet shop and waited until it opened at ten. Red's first thought was to buy another blue and green parakeet, but when they discussed the specifics, they realized that the plan would fail, because a new bird, even if they gave him a crash course would never be able to master Pretty Boy's extensive vocabulary let alone his bodily functions repertoire.

They considered telling Carolyn that he lost his voice because of the cold, but then they would still have the issue of the chipped beak to deal with. Apparently this bird had attempted to mate with himself in a mirror one day and managed to chip his beak in the process. No, the replacement plan wouldn't work—or would it.

They met the pet shop owner as he came to open the store.

"Got any dead birds for sale?" Red asked.

As luck would have it, he did, and for a quarter, they purchased an almost look alike. After they explained the situation, the proprietor even clipped a small piece out of the beak.

They found an empty small red Valentine's Heart candy box, lined it with some velvet from Al's mom's sewing scrap box and dug a hole, with great effort, in Carolyn's back yard. They rang the bell and invited her and her mom to the service. It was a closed casket memorial, but they did flash it open just long enough for Carolyn and Mrs. Primmet to see that the chip was on the wrong side and the colors weren't even close. The two women looked at each other with a look that only two women can give each other and only when they are communicating non-verbally about the stupidity of men, but at that moment, and to this day, they let the boys believe that they pulled it off.

Later that day, Mrs. Primmet explained to Carolyn how sweet it was for her friends to go to all that trouble to try to make her feel better. She also silently hoped that they hadn't started out with a live bird. Carolyn, who didn't really need the explanation, forgave them for letting the bird out in the first place, but she made them each pay three dollars for a new one.

As he drove past a cemetery, Dackel's temporary escape into old memories suddenly exploded like a popped balloon, and his mind, once again, felt the weight of a dead patient who would still be alive if he had only followed his own rule and stayed within the boundaries of his expertise. He had patients die before, but this was the first one he'd killed. He didn't even know how he killed her, but he knew that he was the surgeon and he wasn't in control of his tools and now she's dead.

Dackel wasn't usually the kind of guy who worried about getting sued, but his mind suddenly took him there. He decided that if he did get sued, he would call his insurance carrier and tell them that it was his fault and he did not want to fight it. He would instruct them to write a check for the two hundred thousand policy limit and instruct Pennsylvania's catastrophic loss fund, the holder of his million-dollar umbrella policy, to do the same.

He drove around for hours on the snow-covered roads until he suddenly realized that it was almost time for his weekly meeting with Deborah Metzger-Minkman. There was no way he felt like doing media training that night but he was just a few miles from her office, so he decided to stop up for a minute and tell her that he would have to cancel. Besides, he wanted to see her. He didn't admit to himself why.

He parked the car at a meter that he fed with five quarters, an hour and fifteen minutes worth. As soon as she saw him she knew something was wrong. She closed the door and asked,

"What happened?"

"I had some trouble in the operating room today and I lost a patient, he said.

"Lost like died?" she asked, opening her eyes wide and bringing her hands together in front of her chest, almost as if she was protecting herself from the answer.

"Yep," he said with a deep sigh, "lost, like I killed her."

"How did it happen?" she asked, now with tears in her eyes.

"To tell you the truth, I don't even know. I was using that DAC machine for the first time. The guy who was supposed to be there never came, something happened, and she's dead. I guess I'll find out why tomorrow when they do the post."

"Post?"

"Post-mortem, you know the autopsy."

"Al, what can I do for you?"

"There's nothing to do Deborah. Not a fucking thing to do." Then he thought for a moment and said, "Yeah, there is one thing you can do. You can cancel all those television and radio interviews because you can be damn sure I'm never going to touch that machine again."

Deborah, for the first time in a long time, didn't know what to say and really didn't know what to do. She was used to dealing with damage control. She had taught a supermarket manager how to respond to reporters when the Department of Licenses and Inspections found a dead rat under the meat counter. She helped the operator of a small charter airline defend himself when the press did an exposé on falsified airplane inspection reports. But in those cases, nobody died and in those cases, she hadn't grown quite so fond of her client. She thought for a minute and then got herself together.

"Al, did the TV crew get this on tape?"

"They were there, I guess so," he replied, not realizing the importance of his answer.

She didn't even respond. She just picked up the phone and dialed her best friend Sharon, the executive producer of "Morning in Philly."

"Shar, it's Deb."

"She lets her call her Deb," Dackel thought, still not realizing the potential grenade he was carrying in the hip pocket of his reputation.

"You have to kill the piece." He watched her listen and shake her head from side to side.

"I know, I know, but you can't run it and you can't let news get a hold of it, especially that obnoxious 'ConsumerMan to the Rescue' jerk." She listened again.

"Sharon, if this goes, it will absolutely ruin a good friend of mine. I can't let it happen. I just can't. Who has the tapes? Good, keep them."

"Good friend?" Dackel thought, "She considers me a good friend." For a smart man, sometimes Dackel didn't even see the trees for the trees.

"Shar, I'm asking as a friend—I'm begging as a friend. Give me the tapes. I can't let you ruin this man's life. He's going through too much as it is." She waited what seemed like a very long time. He couldn't read her face. Finally, she smiled, but just a bit.

"Thank you Sharon, I promise that I'll repay you somehow someday. You're a good person. I'll be by in about an hour to pick up the tapes. I don't want them to get into the wrong hands."

"Al, you may not know it, but at this particular moment, I may very well be your best friend."

He knew it. They talked for almost an hour. Dackel just kept going over the same things again and again. She asked a few questions, but mainly, she let him talk. At one point he said something about "this together with all my other troubles." She tilted her head and asked,

"What other troubles?"

He responded, "Oh, you know, this managed care thing, and just life in general, and a new twist, a kid from Florida who is trying to shake me down."

She looked at him questioningly. He told her the whole story, with no sign of embarrassment when he talked about the nudie bar. Perhaps he didn't see her eyebrows rise to the middle of her scalp.

"But I didn't do anything. All I tried to do was help her. I swear," he said, "and I can't figure out what she is going to send me that will make me change my mind. I guess I'll just have to wait and see."

"Al, do you have a good lawyer?"

"What do I need a lawyer for? She wants money. I'm not going to give it to her, and if she bothers me, I'll call the cops. It's as simple as that."

"Poor naive man," thought Deborah, but she said, "Don't make any decisions without talking to me, please."

They talked for another half-hour and left the office together. She went to the television station, he went home.

Metzger-Minkman sat in the editing booth with her forever friend and onetime lover, Sharon Schier. Their relationship had been a lot of different things over the years. Neither considered herself a lesbian, and Deborah felt that she wasn't even bisexual anymore, but they still loved each other as friends. They watched the chaos on the monitor. Neither understood what the hysteroscope camera was showing, but they both realized that footage of the O.R. made it clear that, other than Geller, no one knew what they were doing.

"Debbie, killing this goes against every professional and ethical instinct I have. Not only could I get this on Sixty Minutes, I could expose the whole medical equipment industry. I bet I would wind up saving lives by breaking this story, and my thinking is, if I have to sacrifice one arrogant gynecologist in the process, so be it."

Deborah started to cry. "He's not arrogant, he's very nice. He's just a little boy who never learned the social graces. Besides, I'm asking for my sake as much as I'm asking for his."

"Hey, girlfriend, are you sweet on this guy?" asked Sharon.

"No, not at all," said Deborah, "I just like him and I feel sorry for him. He's caught in a whole handful of messes at this moment and I just want to help him." She cried again.

"Only for you," said Sharon, hugging Deborah tightly. They both felt the love, but neither felt any of the sex that was once there. Sharon ejected the two tapes and handed them to Deborah. They hugged again and Deborah left.

Deborah still had a few tears left to get rid of but she saved them until she got into her car. She thought how lucky she was to have kept Sharon as a friend after their physically intimate relationship ended 6 years ago.

Deborah had grown up in the sixties. At age sixteen she thrust her virginity upon an immature and unprepared junior prom date who that night, couldn't have been happier or more surprised if Ed McMahon himself had come to his door in the Publisher's Clearinghouse Prize Van. (This could never actually have happened since Ed McMahon works for American Family Publishers, so you can imagine how really happy and surprised he was.)

From that night on, she lived an aggressively active sex life, not always being as careful as she could have been, but fortunately being extremely lucky. Deborah liked sex and decided that she should have it whenever she wanted it.

Her marriage had been one of almost unnatural passion and sensuality and the day it was torn asunder by a single 9 mm. bullet, so was her sex drive.

For a long time after her husband's death Deborah didn't even masturbate and didn't even care. Her short sexual relationship with Sharon was only moderately physically rewarding and extremely emotionally uncomfortable. When it ended, Deborah was left with no detectable libido. Eventually, when her sexual needs started to resurface, she did her best to ignore them. Once they became too strong to resist it didn't take her long to remember how good she was at pleasuring herself. The difference was that now, every time she did so, it made her cry.

Still, there was no emotional room for a man. She once confessed to Sharon that she wished there was a service that would send to her house a disease free man with a bag over his head who would come in, not say a word, screw the shit out of her and leave. What she didn't know is that services like that are indeed available.

When Dackel arrived home that evening, Arlene was waiting for him, pacing the floor.

"Al, I'm aggravated, Al," she said in a high clipped tone. "The cleaning service sent someone today who had such a bad body odor that I threw her out. Then they refused to send anyone else. What am I supposed to do. I never should have fired that Martha. It was worth it having to pick her up at the train. Now she took a job with the McDaniel's and I'm stuck. How can I handle this big house by myself. I don't want to have to start with a new service. That means I have to be home..."

"Arlene, I lost a patient on the table today," he said looking at the floor.

"Oh Al, that's terrible. What happened, was it that new machine that you went to Texas for? Is that..."

"Yes, it was during an ablation with the DAC-III, and I don't know what happened, but she died, and I'm responsible."

"Oh Al, you probably didn't do anything, it was probably the machine, you know how new machines are. Remember when we first got the dishwasher and I got a shock because something wasn't connected right? It was probably something like that..."

She was trying the best she knew how to comfort her husband. She just didn't know how. After almost thirty years with him she still couldn't figure out that all he needed was a hug. He told her he needed some time to himself and he went into the family room and shut the door. He sat down in his recliner and just stared at the ceiling. He wished that he could call a service that would send someone over to fall asleep in his arms.

Chapter 22

Dackel hadn't attended an autopsy since freshman anatomy, but this was his first intra-operative death and he felt he should be there. The smell of the morgue brought back memories of medical school. In those days, it wasn't cool to wear gloves during anatomy lab. He dissected his cadaver with his bare hands which smelled from formaldehyde from the first day of class until well into the following August. As soon as he walked in, the chemicals burned his eyes and choked him. The pathologist was an unfriendly fellow about ten years older than Dackel. He had a long, dour face that looked like it belonged to someone who worked with the dead. He nodded to Dackel and pulled back the sheet. He dictated into a microphone suspended above his head.

"This is Dr. Abner Vilsmeier, designated pathologist for the autopsy of Linda Shintock. This autopsy is being performed in the Pathology Department of 14th Street Hospital. In attendance is Dr. Alfred Dackel, the attending physician at the time of the patient's demise."

"The decedent developed a cardiac arrest during a hysteroscopic endometrial ablation and was not able to be resuscitated. On external examination, the body is unclothed. It is the body of a well developed well nourished white female weighing 138 pounds and measuring five feet six inches. Her appearance is consistent with the stated age. Hair and eyes are brown. The conjunctiva and eyelids are edematous. There is bloody mucus seen at both nostrils. The breasts are normal. There are circular defibrillator marks on the right upper chest and left lower chest. The pubic hair is recently shaved. There is bloody fluid in the area of the vagina. The external examination is otherwise normal."

Vilsmeier picked up a scalpel and made an incision across the scalp, which he then peeled back from the skull.

"Reflection of the scalp reveals an intact skull with no evidence of fracture or contusion."

He picked up a saw and sawed off the top of the skull. He made a few cuts with a scalpel and removed the brain and placed it in a scale.

"The brain weighs 1385 grams. There are no signs of hemorrhage, but edema is present."

He made another incision in the neck and exposed the structures.

"The structures of the neck including the thyroid appear normal." The next incision was from the rib cage to the pubic bone. Vilsmeier went on to describe and weigh all of Linda's organs. They all were normal, but many of them, especially the lungs, were swollen with fluid, or as he described them "edematous."

"The uterus shows no signs of perforation." Dackel breathed a sigh of relief. At least her death wasn't due to anything he did wrong. "The uterine muscle shows a five millimeter round defect measuring four millimeters in depth. No thermal effects are noted grossly."

"A five by four millimeter round defect?" he repeated.

"Yes," answered Vilsmeier, "do you know what caused it?"

"No," said Dackel, partly because he wasn't really sure and partly because he really was.

Vilsmeier finished the dictation and told Dackel that he would let him know when the blood analysis and microscopic were done. Dackel thanked him and left the lab wondering how such a small defect could have killed his patient.

The package from Carrie came the next day by UPS. It was a video tape. He waited until his hours were over and his staff was gone. He put it in the VCR and pushed play. He didn't believe what he saw but he especially didn't believe what he heard.

The first scene of the tape showed what looked like someone's living room, but Dackel recognized it as the VIP room at Scampers. It showed him hugging what looked like a high school girl complete with uniform and blond pigtails. The camera was to his back, but he could hear himself saying, "I'm Dr. Alfred Dackel. I can't believe I paid three hundred bucks. I want you. It then switched to a scene of him on the couch with the blond moving up and down between his legs. This was shot from her back, and although you couldn't see very much of him other than his face, it looked like she was performing fellatio on him. There was music in the background, but you could clearly hear him say, "It looks like I wet my pants. Why don't just you give me a pair of panties."

As he watched he was frozen, except for his intestines. His mouth hung open, his eyes didn't blink. The next scene was shot through the window at Denny's. It showed Dackel holding hands across the table with what looked like another girl, this one with short brown hair and wearing a sweatshirt.

The scene changed again, this time to Carrie's apartment. She was standing there naked with a robe at her feet. Alfred was touching her breast. He heard himself saying, "Give me some breasts. They're nice and big, wonderful. Just hold onto it for a second while I unzip."

The picture changed to Dackel hugging a naked Carrie.

The next scene was Carrie lying on the couch and Dackel, shot from the back again, apparently rubbing her pubic area. The only sound was Carrie moaning and telling him, "faster, harder."

But the final scene actually made him ill. It showed Carrie sitting on the toilet with Dackel appearing to be bending over and watching. Fade to black.

He was beside himself. He went into the bathroom and had explosive diarrhea. He was nauseated, and his head ached. He was hoping he would have a heart attack and die on the spot. He didn't. He cleaned himself up and went back to his consultation room. The monitor displayed television snow and white noise came from the speaker. He walked to the phone in slow motion and tried to call Red who had already left his office, was not in his car and not at home. He tried to think but he couldn't. He knew he would not be able to go home in this state, but he had nowhere else to go. Dackel dialed Deborah Metzger-Minkman.

"Deborah, I could really use a friend. Are you busy?"

"Not especially," she said, I just have to drop Emma off at a friend's house for a sleepover. What's the pr*aaaa*blem?"

He no longer heard the nasal whine in her voice. It was still there, of course, he just didn't pay attention to it.

"Remember the girl in Tampa? Well, she sent me this tape and it's bullshit but it looks bad and..."

"Where are you Al?"

"I'm in my office."

"Come on over."

"To your office?" he asked.

"No, come to my apartment."

She gave him the address and he started out the door, hesitating for a second and wondering if she had any hidden cameras anywhere.

When he got there she was wearing a long loose fitting flowered dress, or was it a nightgown? No it was a dress, but she may not have been wearing a bra. Those thoughts flashed through his mind as if they were required to, despite their inappropriateness at the time. They walked toward each other as if they were going to hug, but they both stopped a few feet short of contact. He thanked her for inviting him and handed her the tape.

"Before you watch this, I want you to understand that this is not what happened. He explained what she was about to see. "The voice is mine, but I didn't say those things." He told her that he figured out that somehow, Carrie got a hold of tapes from the security system at Scampers and she also must have had her apartment bugged. But where did the voice come from? It sounded like him, but he certainly didn't remember saying those things, or did he?

He played the tape for her. He could tell she was shocked. Again, he explained what really went on and she believed him. They played the tape again and wrote down everything he said.

"I want you to try to remember whether you said any of this stuff—anywhere.

"I'm Dr. Alfred Dackel." He did say that in the club. He remembered introducing himself to Carrie, who at the time, he thought was Angel.

"I can't believe I paid three hundred bucks." "Three hundred bucks, he didn't recall saying anything about three hundred bucks— except—when he was making the tape at National, he was talking about his glasses and he did remember making reference to the fact that they cost three hundred bucks. But how did she get that tape?

"I want you." That didn't even sound right.

"That sounds funny," said Deborah. "I would have expected that you would have dropped your voice after 'you.' But instead, it sounds like your sentence was cut off in the middle. 'I want you,'" she said over and over. Then it hit her. She ejected Carrie's tape and put in the patient information tape that he made at the meeting. She had a copy which she had planned to send to the medical reporters on the news shows.

"Hello, I'm Dr. Alfred Dackel, and I want you to meet a good friend of mine, Dr. Mark MacDonald." The "I want you" matched perfectly and so did the "I'm Dr. Alfred Dackel."

It was obvious that Carrie had gotten a hold of the tape. He went down the list of quotes.

"It looks like I wet my pants." He remembered saying that when he spilled the water on himself while he was getting ready to make the tape. He also remembered saying "Why don't just you give me a pair of panties," when he saw himself in makeup.

"Give me some breasts. They're nice and big, wonderful." He remembered saying the first part when he was getting made up for the video and he also remembered that the TelePrompTer letters were nice and big, but that was also before he started the tape.

"Just hold onto it for a second while I unzip." The only thing he remembered unzipping was the garment bag when they gave him his shirt for the taping.

It was obvious that Carrie had access not only to the patient education tape, but also all the raw footage. She had to have a link to National Medical. Dackel guessed it was Donny Moline.

"Al, I believe you. I can tell that this tape was edited. There are differences in the background noises. Each room has its own sound. It's because of the air conditioner, the traffic, the rugs and drapes and even the height of the ceiling. There are at least two different room noises here. Besides, some of the edits are not quite perfect. This tape is definitely bogus."

Dackel wondered how much Arlene knew about room noises and edits.

"I think you ought to call the cops, Al. She's shaking you down," said Deborah.

"Let me think about it," he said as he left her apartment.

Dackel called Carrie the next day and told her that he needed some time to think. He really did. She told him she would give him two weeks.

As soon as he hung up, Vilsmeier called.

"I just got the lab tests back on Shintock," he said without any "hello" or "how are you." "Her sodium was very low and so was her serum osmolality. These are both signs of water intoxication. I checked with the anesthesia record and Geller was using Plasmalyte and he didn't use that much of it so it couldn't have been anything he did. What were you putting through your hysteroscope?"

Dackel froze. He had heard the words water intoxication at the course. He knew what it was. Blood has to contain a certain number of "particles," like sodium, potassium and chloride. If there are not enough particles, or if the particles aren't in balance, major problems can occur. The central nervous system, the heart, the kidneys and the blood can all be effected. The bottom line is that if water intoxication is not recognized and treated promptly, death can occur. Apparently it did. But why did she become water intoxicated?

"Dr., are you still there?" asked Vilsmeier.

"Yes, I was just thinking," replied Dackel.

Vilsmeier continued, "My guess is that that small defect I saw was in the area of some major blood vessels. I suspect that the distending fluid was forced into the vascular system by pressure from the pump. But even so, most distending solutions shouldn't cause water intoxication. What did you use to distend the uterus? It wasn't noted on the nurses notes."

Dackel didn't know what to do. He still wasn't sure that water was the wrong thing to use, but it was sounding more and more like it was.

"I don't know what she used," he said, putting the responsibility on the nurse. "I'll check it out and get back to you."

Dackel immediately went to his bookcase and found the packet from the Tampa course. He looked for a section on distending solutions in the monograph that he had never really read through.

"The following media have been used for uterine distention during hysteroscopy," it read, "carbon dioxide, physiologic saline, glycine, sorbitol, mannitol, high molecular weight dextran..." He stopped reading the list when he saw the sentence that began the next paragraph.

"Under no circumstances should hypo-osmolar fluids such as plain water be used. Because of it's hypotonicity, absorption into the circulatory system can result in water intoxication and potential fatality."

Dackel called the operating room. Anna Nichols was gone for the day. He called the nursing service department to get her home phone number.

"Anna, this is Dr. Dackel."

"Hi Dr. Dackel, are you okay?" she asked sincerely.

"Anna, you know how these things affect us all. It's rough."

"I know," she said sympathetically.

"Anna, I'm sorry to interrupt you at home, but do you, by any chance, remember what kind of fluid we used to distend Mrs. Shintock's uterus?"

"I remember we were looking at a few different options, but to be honest with you, Dr. Dackel, I don't remember which one you handed me. I just hung it."

"Thanks Anna," said Dackel, letting out a big breath after he hung up. This was a dilemma for Dackel. He was basically an honest person, but if he told the truth and admitted that he used sterile water despite the fact that the literature warned against it, he could be in big trouble. For the first time in his life, Dackel thought seriously about suicide. He called Vilsmeier's office and left a message that he didn't remember which solution was used. Maybe Anna Nichols remembered.

Dackel went to the hospital library and found a book on complications of hysteroscopy. There was a chapter on water intoxication. As he read, he felt sicker and sicker.

"The intravascular absorption of a hypotonic irrigation fluid is one of the most serious complications of hysteroscopic procedures. The fluid used for irrigation enters the circulation through the vascular spaces opened during the procedure. Occasionally, an injury or tear in the lower uterine segment from dilation, or perforation of the uterus may expose large vascular channels..."

He now knew exactly what happened. Dimucci fell against the DAC-III hitting the test buttons. The DAC fired a test pulse that made the small defect in the endometrium. It bled a little obscuring his view so he turned up the pressure of the sterile water. The water entered her circulation and diluted her blood, lowering her sodium concentration enough to kill her. He was responsible. He did it. He should have known better. He wondered who else was going to figure this out.

Chapter 23

Two weeks later Carrie Bradford called. Dackel didn't return the call. He hadn't done any constructive thinking about her demands or the tape. He hid it in his office but he kept moving it because he was afraid his hiding places weren't good enough. As he was putting it up above a ceiling tile, his secretary buzzed him to tell him there was someone to see him. He went out to his waiting room and said hello to an attractive woman who introduced herself as Merri Pucat. She asked if he was Alfred Dackel and when he responded affirmatively she handed him an envelope. He thanked her and opened it getting what seemed like a potentially fatal paper cut in the process. An official looking document read:

Court of Common Pleas

> **You have been sued in court. If you wish to defend against the claims set forth in the following pages, you must take action within 20 days after this complaint notice...**"

Next to "Plaintiffs" were the names Paul Shintock and The Estate of Linda Shintock (deceased). The defendants were listed as Alfred P. Dackel, M.D., Arnold A. Geller, M.D., Fourteenth Street Hospital, Anna Nichols, R.N., National Medical Innovations, and John Doe, just in case they found someone else with insurance who waved to the patient at any time during her hospital stay.

Dackel expected that he would get sued, but that didn't prevent his stomach from twisting when he opened the notice. He had been sued before, but those times it had been different because he knew he hadn't done anything wrong. One case was a woman who didn't like the way her Caesarian scar healed. He won that case. Another was a woman who came to him because she was unable to get pregnant. She claimed that the medication he gave her made her worse. Although he couldn't understand how you can make infertility worse with a fertility medicine that didn't work, his lawyer convinced him to settle the case settled for nuisance value. He had also been also sued by a woman who claimed that she lost her psychic powers after he tied her tubes. The jury awarded her 1.2 million, but it was thrown out on appeal.

Dackel called his insurance company and asked to speak to the claims representative. Of course, no one was available, but he was told to fax a copy of the papers. Later that day he got a call from the law firm of Dagget, Laurel, Stratton, Binsley & Rittenhouse.

"Dr. Dackel, this is Stacey Finney, I'll be your attorney on the Shintock case. I need you to send me all of your records regarding Ms. Shintock and also copies of all the bills and payments..."

"Wait a minute," interrupted Dackel, "just wait a minute. I don't want a lawyer. I was trying to tell the insurance company to give Paul Shintock whatever he wants. I know it was my fault. I never should have done the operation to begin with."

"Dr. Dackel, your carrier assigns every case to an attorney, even the ones that settle. Please, just let me look at the records and we can sit down and talk about it. You know, you're not the only one named in this suit and not everyone is likely to agree with you about how to resolve it. And quite frankly, it's not up to you. It's up to your insurance carrier. I need to meet with you to get some details. I've subpoenaed the records but it would help if you bring me copies of everything you have."

"I want this resolved," said Dackel, "I'll come tomorrow at four. Where's your office?"

"I can't make it tomorrow. I can see you next Thursday at three," she replied tersely, not because she really couldn't see him tomorrow, but because she wanted to show him who was running the show.

He went home that night hoping that Arlene would be out. It was not that he didn't like her. He did, but tonight he needed the kind of emotional support and nurturing that she was incapable of providing. Arlene was a good person but she was so self-absorbed that there wasn't much left for anyone else. All these years he didn't even know what he was missing. He realized it only recently, partly because of his relationship with Deborah and partly, believe it or not, because of things that came out in his sessions with Capuston. He also realized that he too was kind of short in the support-giving department.

Arlene was home. He tried, once again, to talk about their relationship.

"Arlene, Paul Shintock is suing me. The lawyer who's going to represent me called today." he started.

"Is he a good lawyer Al?" she asked.

"It's a she. The lawyer is a woman," he answered, "and I don't know if she's good. She sounds young. Arlene, I'm really upset about this case."

"Oh, I'm sure everything will be okay. The trial won't interfere with our trip to Boca, will it Al?" she asked.

"Arlene, I don't know when the trial is, it might not come up for three years."

"Well how are we supposed to plan our vacations? Can't you get them to tell you at least what month it will be?"

"Yeah, I'll try," said Dackel, realizing that he couldn't make her what she wasn't, "I'll try."

The following Thursday, Dackel walked five blocks from his office to the offices of Dagget, Laurel, Stratton, Binsley & Rittenhouse. They were on the twelfth floor of a brand new office building in front of which was a sculpture that looked to him like a huge pile of dog crap. Philadelphia had passed a law requiring anyone who built a new commercial building to spend a percentage of the total cost on some sort of exterior artwork. This particular monsterpiece must have been chosen to get back at city council.

The receptionist had what he called bubble hair. It looked like someone inflated it with a bicycle pump. She did have a low cut blouse though, and when she got up to take his coat, he saw that she was wearing a short leather skirt and the shiny kind of stockings that he liked. She told him to have a seat until Ms. Finney was ready for him.

Ms. Finney looked like she was a seventeen-year-old dressed in her mommy's clothes. Of course she wore a blue business suit and a fashionably unoriginal white silk blouse. All women lawyers did. She was cute in a high school kind of way and actually reminded him of his latest object of hatred, Carrie Bradford.

"Hi Dr. Dackel, I'm Stacey Finney. We spoke on the phone and I think I might have gone to summer camp with your son. Was his name Brant or something?"

"Yes," he said, "Brent was my son."

"I'm really sorry, he was really cool."

"Yes, he was," said Dackel, hating the fact that he was once again forced to think about the call from the police and the frantic ride to the hospital to identify his only child's shredded body still dressed in the remnants of his senior prom tuxedo. The drunk who hit him, a Catholic priest, served three months and lost his drivers license for a year.

Dackel pushed the memory from his mind, knowing full well that it would be back some night—soon.

"Look, Miss Finney, like I said on the phone, I don't want to go to court on this thing. She died and I'm responsible and it was because I really didn't know what I was..."

"Stop Dr. Dackel! Don't say anything else. Just listen to me. Hypothetically, if a complication arose during an operation and that complication was a direct cause of a death, and a doctor's negligence was somehow responsible for that complication, then a case like that will either settle or it will try, and that doctor will tell the jury just what happened. But if, and this is still hypothetical, the doctor were to testify that he knew going into this case that he or she had not been qualified to do the operation, the best case is that the doctor could be required to pay punitive damages, maybe in the millions, that may not be covered by malpractice insurance. And that's the best scenario."

"If that's the best..." interrupted Dackel.

"Uh-uh, don't talk yet. The worst case is that the doctor could be tried criminally for manslaughter. That could mean jail. So, before you say anything, I want you to realize that if the circumstances in the Shintock case are anything like the hypothetical example I just gave you, you might be in some heavy-duty trouble. Now let's you and I talk about the Shintock case, and from this point on, I am the only one you talk to—not your friends, not your family, just me. Got it?"

"Yes," he answered with his head down. Dackel wasn't even good at blustering anymore. Not only was medicine passing him by, but it seemed that the whole world was.

"The plaintiff's attorney is Sylvan Sheldon," she continued. "His philosophy is that he yells and screams and gets as much publicity as he can. He doesn't have a whole lot in the way of ethics and he's not a nice guy. He will do everything he can to ruin you. You also have to know that he is very successful at what he does and he doesn't usually take a case unless he's fairly confident that he will score big. Now I want you to tell me everything about your care of Linda Shintock and everything about the DAC-III, starting from the beginning, and just the facts—no opinions, no interpretations."

He spent the next two hours telling her what she needed to know. He left out the part about the sterile water. Whenever he started to say, "I think," or "I feel," she would stop him.

"No opinions yet, Dr. Dackel, just facts." She took notes on long white paper. Dagget, Laurel, Stratton, Binsley & Rittenhouse had long abandoned the customary yellow legal pads. They said that it had something to do with the environment, but it was really because the white ones were cheaper.

He left her office exhausted and depressed. As he walked through the park on the way back to his office, he felt like curling up on a bench and dying, but he figured that with his luck, he'd probably just get shit on by the pigeons.

Two weeks later, Dackel had a really bad day—three bad phone calls and a really bad meeting. The first call was from Red's friend Spencer.

"Hi. Dr. Dackel, Spence Dishay from QHM. Listen, I had this application just about pushed through, but there was a discrepancy. You stated that you didn't have any outstanding law suits, but your insurance carrier says you have a death case pending."

"That's because it was filed after I filled out the application," responded Dackel.

"I realize that, but you initialed the part that said, "If any information on this application changes between now and the time I receive notification of your action with regard to my request for inclusion on your approved physician list, I will notify the QHM immediately of such changes."

"There were twenty different things I initialed. Okay, consider yourself notified. Now when am I going to be reinstated?"

"I'm afraid it's not that easy now," said Dishay, with a very different tone than he had when Red was present, "the committee considers this falsification of credentials."

"That's total bullshit!" Dackel screamed, once again freeing the jerk within, "You guys are a bunch of maggots. Forget it! I need QHM like I need another asshole." He hung up.

Forty minutes later Carrie called.

"Hi Al," she had her hard voice on, "When can I expect my money?"

"Carrie, or whatever your name is, give me a break. I just got sued for malpractice, I got thrown out of my biggest HMO and if my life turned totally to shit, it would be an improvement. I just can't deal with this now. I figured out how you rigged the tape and I'm pretty sure who did it for you. If I hear from you again, I'm going to call the cops. Now leave me alone!" He hung up, naively thinking that he had handled the situation pretty well.

The third call was from Stacey Finney who told him that the Shintock's attorney had added punitive damages to the suit. This meant that he could be financially "punished." In addition to paying compensatory damages, Sheldon would try to show that Dackel was guilty of gross negligence or willful disregard of the consequences. Some states had limits on punitive damages, but unfortunately, Pennsylvania was not one of them.

She also told him that they wanted to schedule a deposition as soon as possible. She explained that a deposition was part of what was called discovery. It meant that the plaintiff's attorney wanted to get information from Dackel that they could use to help formulate their case. She also explained that the deposition was sworn testimony and anything that he said could turn around and "bite him in the ass" during the trial. It was therefore important that he be intimately familiar with the records and that they meet before the actual deposition to "straighten out a few facts." What she really meant was that they would go over the answers to the questions that she figured they would ask. They set up an appointment for Thursday afternoon, after he finished his surgery.

That same day, Jerry Edmonds returned from Europe. He had heard about Dackel's patient and the lawsuit during his daily telephone updates. He went right from the airport to the executive conference room at National Medical Innovations. The room was a richly appointed, comfortable room. At the moment, no one was comfortable. MacDonald and Clark were waiting for him. The three of them who were all smiles at the course were, right now, all business. Jerry Edmonds was pacing impatiently while Donny Moline was fiddling with the video monitor.

"This could fucking ruin us," he said with venom dripping from each word, "I knew this guy was trouble from the beginning. We never should have given him a machine, and we absolutely never should have left him on his own." He glared at MacDonald who sat slumped at the mirror finished oak conference table. "The first patient in phase two testing of the DAC-III dies. Do we know why she died? Does anyone know why she died? MacDonald, do you know why she died?"

"I-I'm not sure. There was confusion, and I didn't see part of the feed because they lost their monitor, and..."

"I blame you for this, you know. You should have told him to hold the operation 'till you got there," said Edmonds glaring at MacDonald.

MacDonald passed on the glare to Cal Clark who dropped his eyes. He was hoping that MacDonald wouldn't let it be known that it was he who pushed him into pushing Dackel to operate. MacDonald didn't say anything, but swore to himself the moment he felt that his job was in jeopardy, he would sing like Ethel Merman.

"Donny, what's holding up the tape?" Edmonds said with a slow burn.

"Ready to go sir."

"Well then let's go!" whined Edmonds impatiently.

They watched as the tape showed a very calm typical operating room scene. The patient was smiling and happy. The nurses were busy readying the equipment, hooking up the fluid to distend the uterus during the hysteroscopy, test firing the DAC-III, laying out the hysteroscopy set. They saw Dackel sit down between the patient's legs and insert the speculum into the vagina and the scope into the uterus. They saw the split screen image of a normal operating room on the left side of the screen and the inside of a normal uterus on the right. They listened as Dackel asked Dimucci if he could see and watched as Dimucci tripped while moving to get a better view. That was the point where he pulled out the monitor cord and all hell broke loose but the tape continued to record both pictures.

"Wait a minute, run that back, and play it again in slow motion," said MacDonald. Donny rewound the last few seconds and played it at one forth the normal speed.

"Look at that, that was a flash in the uterus. The DAC fired, he said. Run it back again, slower. This time go frame by frame." Donny did. Okay, look at that frame, That's the flash, do you see it?" Everyone agreed. "Now look at the left side of the screen. Do you see it? The resident- he falls against the machine with both hands. The son of a bitch hit the test fire buttons. Jesus Christ, we put them far apart so they wouldn't be fired by accident. What are the odds?"

"Doesn't matter what the odds were," said Edmonds, "whatever they were, we lost."

"The patient lost," said MacDonald under his breath.

"Why did she die?" asked Clark.

Edmonds glared at him.

"Let's go frame by frame after the test fire," said MacDonald. "Look, the bleeding is starting from the lateral aspect of the cavity. That's where the uterine arteries are. But the test fire shouldn't have gone that deep, unless the scope was right up against the wall. Go back to the frames just before the flash, right after the kid trips. Okay, he trips-now look, Dackel turns to see what the noise was, and as he turns—look at the other side of the screen now—as he turns, he moves the scope right into the wall. Look, you can see it. Donny keep going back and forth—do you see?"

"I still don't understand," said Clark, "I thought this thing only hits targeted tissue."

"It does when it's in the 'treat' mode," said MacDonald, " but in the test mode, it targets a five by four millimeter circle of whatever it encounters. That, combined with the fact that the scope was directly over the vessels, caused a nice chunk to be vaporized. I don't think it hit the uterine artery, but it definitely opened up a few vessels. That's where the bleeding is coming from. But that's not enough bleeding to kill her. I'm sure of that."

"Well it doesn't matter what you're sure of, I'm sure that regardless of why she died, we're going to take it up the ass with the FDA's boot," said Edmonds. This cannot be a hysteroscopy-related death. MacDonald, could the anesthesiologist have screwed up? If it was an anesthesia death, they can't blame us."

"I don't know, Jerry, it could have been," said MacDonald, "but the test fire, I mean it looks pretty incriminating, and if they question Dackel about his experience, we're dead."

"What did the autopsy show?" asked Edmonds

"We should have it by this afternoon," answered MacDonald.

"Then we'll talk this afternoon. Donny, I'd like to see to you in my office in a half-hour."

In the two years he worked at National, Donny had never been in Edmond's office. He was worried that he took too much time setting up the video, and also a little worried that someone caught on to some of the after hours work he was doing with the company's equipment. He was wrong about both.

"Donny," Edmonds said, sounding like a godfather on his death bed, "I have worked very hard to bring the DAC-III to market. Most of my time and all of my money have been spent perfecting this machine. It's a good machine. It just got into the wrong hands, and it's unfair that that one error, and it was our error, might ruin us. I'm going to say something that I don't want you to respond to. In fact, I don't want you to say anything at all about it, now or ever." Edmonds took a thick envelope out of his pocket and slipped it into Donny's breast pocket.

"I'm not as sure as the others that I saw that flash or the test fire buttons being pushed. Thanks for coming up here, Donny." Edmonds swiveled his high-backed leather chair 180 degrees and stared out the window until Donny left the room.

Jerry Edmonds was always a star who managed to screw up. He had the highest grades in his M.B.A. program at The Wharton School, but he never bothered to write his thesis so he never got his degree. Despite that he got a job with a large pharmaceutical company and rapidly advanced to national sales manager. That was about the time that the government started to investigate bribery in the industry and, although he never went to jail, he made a very convenient scapegoat and was fired for the press release value.

Being a survivor, he started a small company of his own and with a combination of brains, contacts and unscrupulous business practices, he built it into what it now was. One thing for sure was that he was not going to let this incident derail him.

Donny went back to his control room and opened the envelope. There was a thick stack of hundred dollar bills inside, fifty of them. He put them in his pocket, popped in the tape and worked his magic. He put the original master in his brief case and dropped two copies of the new tape on the receptionist's desk in the executive suite.

Jerry called his pilot and told him to fuel up the Lear and file a flight plan for Philadelphia. He picked up a copy of the tape and the just-arrived autopsy report to review on the plane and had his driver take him to the airport. They were there by three. His secretary had called ahead and arranged a meeting with Dackel in his office at six. They got to Dackel's office just as he was finishing up.

"Dr. Dackel, I heard about the unfortunate complication your patient experienced, and I want to help," said Edmonds with his charm once again turned on.

"Can you raise the dead?" asked Dackel sarcastically.

"No, but I can offer the services of National Medical Innovations' legal department to help you get through this as painlessly as possible. From what I understand, the plaintiff's attorney is very loud but not too smart. We may be able to convince him to take a settlement with a confidentiality clause. Face it, someone's going to pay for this death. The goal now is to keep your reputation and the reputation of National Medical Innovations and the DAC-III from being destroyed."

"That's fine with me," replied Dackel. "I want to settle it."

"It would really be better for us if they let National out of the suit early. One of the ways you could help us is to make sure you get a few statements in during your deposition. It's important that you say that the machine did not malfunction in any way during the procedure. Also it would be good if you mentioned that we were not aware that you were not an experienced hysteroscopist. And lastly, it would be better if the whole MacDonald thing wasn't mentioned at all."

"Are you crazy?" yelled Dackel. I'm not about to purger myself so that you get out of trouble and I get in deeper. How stupid do you think I am!"

"Let me finish," said Edmonds. "We've invested a great deal of money in this instrument and we hope it will earn us all a lot of money. We're also convinced that it's safe and easy to use. This was an unfortunate accident, but it could ruin us. We are willing to support your legal defense in every way, and we will even personally guarantee any punitive damages you may incur."

"Will you go to jail for me if they find out I lied?" asked Dackel.

"There should be no reason anyone should find out anything," Edmonds answered. "Besides, we reviewed the tape of the operation and we don't see any evidence of mechanical malfunction. In fact, the DAC-III was not even activated at any time during the procedure. The autopsy shows a gouge in the side of the uterus. That could have been trauma from the hysteroscope."

"I'm not going to lie under oath. You guys told me I was ready to use this thing. You guys told me to go ahead without MacDonald, and you guys aren't going to lay this whole thing on me. If you can do anything to get it settled, then do it. I killed this woman. You helped. You hear me?"

Edmonds left the office with somewhat less than his salesman's grace. As soon as he got on the plane, he called the main office and asked for his Pedro Sanchez, National's Director of Corporate Security to met him at the airport. He was there when the plane landed. They got into Sanchez's car, both of them in the front seat.

"Pedro, I need some information on a Dr. Alfred Dackel in Philadelphia. I'd prefer if you would keep this within the family, so why don't you pack a bag and head on down there for a few days and see what you can dig up."

Pedro didn't mess around. He got his training as a covert operative in a country where human rights and civil liberties didn't mean a whole lot. His skills and his lack of conscience were rented by Jerry Edmonds for significant reimbursement. In the company's infancy, Pedro had done some "research" at several other medical technology companies that helped Edmonds with his business plan. Sanchez would manage to get custodial jobs at these companies, jobs that gave him access to two of the most important things in industrial spying, the night and the trash. He was always amazed at how easy it was to come across designs, patent applications and the all-important memo. It also didn't hurt that he was also an expert computer hacker. He was a bulky man with a large thick face and hair that was short on top, but he had a long ponytail that reached to his waist. When he had to look corporate, he just tucked it in the back of his shirt.

When he arrived in Philadelphia the next night, he went straight to Dackel's office building to have a look. No apparent alarm, a sleepy desk man and access to the roof of the building from the parking lot next door. By 1:35 A.M. Dackel's office was bugged. While he was hiding the tape recorder above a ceiling tile, he felt something with his hand. It was a videotape. He took the tape but left the box. He would copy it and return it the next night when he came to pick up the audio tape from his recorder which he had, of course, moved to the other side of the room.

Sanchez checked into a Comfort Inn near the river. He could have afforded the Four Seasons, but he didn't look like he belonged there and he knew it. Actually, even the clerk at the Comfort asked for another form of identification besides his credit card. Sanchez asked if there was a VCR in the room and the clerk just laughed. He could have gone to an all-night video store to rent one, but he decided to go to sleep instead.

When he awoke the next morning he went to the closest K-Mart, purchased two inexpensive VCR's and took them back to his room. He watched the tape as he copied it. He knew the female romantic lead. Even though he heard Dackel call her Carrie, he knew it was Alice Kirkland, Donny Moline's girlfriend. He called Jerry.

At the same time Sanchez was on the phone with Edmonds, Dackel was on the phone with Red. He told him that he wanted to stop seeing Capuston. He had been there the previous evening wasting another hour talking about his mother. He told Red that he was finished. Red convinced him to hang in for a few more sessions.

"With the law suit and this new bullshit with QHM, you have to keep it up. In fact, I'm going to move up our timeline. It's not going to be two years, I want to file soon. I'll prepare the papers. It's simple. I've gone over your disability policy. You are insured as a gynecologic surgeon. It says that you can collect twelve thousand a month if you are unable to perform surgery. Do you realize what that means? It means that you can continue to practice, and see all the patients you want in your office. You can hire another kid to do all of your surgery for you, and you get a guaranteed buck forty four a year just for waking up in the morning. You increase my retainer another twenty for my efforts, and you relax. Two or three years, I'll be ready to retire, you'll be ready to retire, we'll have a ball.

All you have to do is convince the insurance company that you're mentally unfit to operate. Capuston will have to testify that you came to him and said you were afraid even before the whole hysteroscopy thing happened. The death will be the icing on the cake!"

Dackel didn't like the whole thing. He always suspected that Red was a latent crook. It did seem like a foolproof idea though. How could the insurance company prove that he was not afraid to operate—unless of course they got a hold of the phone bug tape that Pedro Sanchez would recover later that day from the recorder that he had stashed in the ceiling.

When he heard tape of Dackel's call to Red, Pedro knew he had all he needed. He could ruin Dackel in two different ways. He called the Lear pilot and told him to be ready in an hour.

After Edmonds talked to Sanchez he realized that he had another problem for which he would need Sanchez's help. He had to figure out how to deal with Donny Moline. The tape established the fact that Donny was an extortionist and Jerry couldn't have that to worry about.

Edmonds was waiting at the airport for Pedro. Larry Ainsley, Director of National's Legal Affairs Department was also in the limo.

"Mr. Sanchez has inadvertently come across some information about Dr. Dackel that we thought you might want to know about, Larry," said Edmonds, feeling his way slowly with Ainsley who had been with the company for less than a year. For most of that year he handled patent issues and contracts. "It seems that Dr. Dackel is planning to commit insurance fraud against his disability carrier. Mr. Sanchez feels that he can document the fact that Dr. Dackel is lying to a psychiatrist in order to create a medical file that shows he has a mental illness that will allow him to collect indefinite disability payments."

"How did you come upon this information, Mr. Sanchez?" asked Ainsley, who showed some interest, but no real excitement.

"Let's just say for now that I believe I can get my hands on a tape recording of a telephone conversation during which he admits the scam to a confidant."

"Well, unless that recording was made during a legal wiretap, or was given to you with the express permission of the confidant, and was made with the knowledge of Dr. Dackel, it's useless," said Ainsley.

Edmonds shook his head as if he were agreeing with Ainsley. He knew what he had to do. He thanked Ainsley for coming and dropped him off at his home. As Ainsley was getting out of the car, he asked Edmonds, probably for the forth time that week, whether he got Linda Shintock's autopsy report. Edmonds lied and said no.

"Do you want me to handle this?" asked Sanchez.

"I don't think so Pedro, not at this point. Get someone from outside the company, but make sure it's someone who can be trusted. Start with the Kirkland tape. Threaten to send it to his wife and the television tabloids, you know, 'Prominent Gynecologist Gets Caught with Teenager' or something like that. If that doesn't work we'll use the disability thing. If nothing works, we'll subpoena this Capuston character and get him to admit in a deposition that Dackel was afraid to operate when he used the DAC-III. But don't do anything yet. I want to get some more information about Sheldon and I also want to get an idea of how quickly this case is progressing. Let's save our ammunition. Now what are we going to do with Donny?" asked Edmonds.

"I don't see what the big deal is," said Sanchez. "So what if he's a scammer?"

With a great deal of reluctance, Edmonds told Sanchez that he had Moline alter the surgery tape.

"You should not have done that Jerry," Sanchez said shaking his head. "You should not have done that without consulting with me. It should never have been done in-house. I could have had it done right by someone I could trust. You never should have done that. The kid's an extortionist. Who knows how many times he's done this? He has you by the balls now."

"Well, it's done," responded Edmonds. "Now what do we do?"

"The first thing is to call off Alice Kirkland. I'll send someone around with a fake FBI badge and warn her that we're on to her and tell her that we'll have her ass in jail for forty years if she contacts Dackel or anyone else. I'll try to get the original tape, but I'm sure Moline has it stashed somewhere. Also, I don't want to tip Alice off that we know Moline's involved."

Pedro called his old acquaintance, Bruce Cosmo. He chose him because he, like Sanchez, was essentially a mercenary whose ethics were for rent. He was tough and scary looking and he knew how to get a job done. He filled him in on the details and when he mentioned Dackel's name, Cosmo didn't even flinch.

Chapter 24

Dackel got the call as he was making rounds at the hospital. Arlene had been in an accident. She was on her way back from her manicurist and her car went out of control and hit a tree. She had a broken leg from where she was thrown against the dashboard but the airbag had protected her head and chest. Dackel left his hospital and sped over to Community General. He knew why it happened. Whenever she got her nails done she had this funny way of driving so they wouldn't get messed up. She would spread all of her fingers apart and drive with her palms. Of course, they might get smeared when she put on her seatbelt, so she never did. He had warned her about it many times.

When he got to the emergency room she was on a transport stretcher about to be transferred to her hospital room. Dackel didn't know the orthopod, a guy by the name of Matt Laffey, but he introduced himself and got the story. Her femur was broken and it would need to be pinned in the morning, but it looked like a pretty routine case and she would be out of the hospital in a few days. The femur or thigh bone is the largest bone in the body and has a great deal of marrow in its core. Sometimes a broken femur can bleed enough that the patient can die. That didn't seem to be the case in this accident. He invited Dackel to observe the surgery, but Dackel declined. He knew that it put pressure on a surgeon to have a family member watching and besides, all that drilling and banging and nailing made him sick.

Arlene was heavily sedated and she only grunted when Al tried to talk to her. He was upset, but not really worried. It could have been worse. She was medicated and would probably sleep for the rest of the night so he kissed her on the head and went home.

The next morning he paced the floor in the surgical family waiting area like a nervous cat. Meanwhile, in O.R. 3, Arlene was laid out on an airplane table, which was so named because it looked like a table with wings. It was used for operating on extremities. Matt Laffey looked at the x-rays hanging in the lighted view box and tugged at Arlene's leg until it was in position. After the leg was prepped and draped, he made a three inch incision, but when he encountered a layer of fat that was thicker than he anticipated, he enlarged it to five inches. He split some of the muscle fibers of her gluteus maximus and exposed the bone. With an awl, he made a pilot hole and then directed a metal Steinman Pin into the marrow cavity of the bone.

The operation went well and when Laffey gave the good news to Dackel, they both seemed relieved. Everyone involved in the medical profession jokes (although no one really thinks it's a joke) that medical people and their families have more complications and medical bad luck than the rest of the world. It looked like Arlene Dackel beat the curse today.

Al drove back to his office with one less thing to worry about. Of course, there was still a hefty list. He thought about his Florida stripper/extortionist at about the same time she was thinking about him.

Alice called Donny at work. "I'm really scared, Donny. The FBI was here today. I'm so scared. Dackel must have reported us."

"That doesn't make sense," said Donny. "He would have to tell them what was on the tape. You know a guy like him wouldn't do that. What did you tell the agent?"

"I didn't say much of anything. He said he was on to me and if I didn't cease and desist from asking for money, he would arrest me."

She didn't tell him the whole story. Bruce Cosmo had come in, flashed a badge, put Kirkland in handcuffs and searched her apartment until he found the tape. He told her that she was under arrest for extortion and would probably go to jail for thirty years. He then told her that he had to strip-search her and perform a body cavity check. After her clothes were off, Alice offered him a deal. He accepted. When they were through, that's when he gave her the warning and let her go.

"Well I don't know what happened," Donny said, "but if they didn't arrest you, you'll probably be okay.

Chapter 25

Stacey Finney called. The Shintock case was moving along rapidly which was unusual. The typical malpractice action took three or four years to come to trial. It looked like this one would be ready in a year. The Shintock's attorneys had scheduled Dackel's deposition in a few weeks. Finney wanted to spend a day with him going over the facts of the case. She also wanted him to be prepared to respond to the media. She fully expected Sylvan Sheldon to leak the case to the press.

Most attorneys feel that it is unethical and even risky to do that, but Sheldon loved the camera. He had taken a course with someone who had taken a course with the media coach who trained the lawyers on the O.J. defense team. He learned some ridiculous things, such as looking over the camera, not into it. Most television people knew that all that did was make you look stupid and it made your head look smaller and your nose bigger. Nonetheless, Sheldon thought Robert Shapiro was the greatest, and like all of the Simpson attorneys, he loved publicity.

Finney suggested that Dackel get some coaching by one Deborah Metzger-Minkman. He told his lawyer he would cooperate fully, but he never got around to calling her. He was busy trying to earn a living, keeping his house in order and visiting his wife in the hospital.

Arlene was lying in her hospital bed in a peignoir ensemble consisting of powder blue satin robe over a coordinating nightgown. The final component to this outfit was a matching wide headband, which looked more like half of a turban. She was probably trying to look like a glamorous movie star from the forties, but she looked ridiculous.

She rang for her nurse who learned to ignore her buzzer until she rang it for the third or fourth time. Arlene seemed to feel that this highly competent, well-trained and very busy medical professional was her personal upstairs maid. So far during her stay, she had summoned her to turn her pillow because it had become hot, to tuck in the bottom of the sheet which had come loose, and to "freshen" the water in her three quarters filled pitcher which had been freshened only an hour earlier.

The best call, the one they are still talking about at Community came at precisely 4:03 P.M. two days after Arlene's surgery, when she feverishly pushed her call button. The nurse answered through the intercom.

"Yes Mrs. Dackel, can I help you?"

"Myra, you must come in here right away. Hurry Myra!"

Although Myra was already used to Arlene, this call did seem urgent. She dropped her clipboard and ran to the room. Arlene was sitting up in bed and staring at the television.

"Myra dear, Oprah has the entire cast of Chicago Hope on today, and I knew you wouldn't want to miss it. You know, you being a nurse and everything."

But this time it was different. Arlene really didn't feel well. She was feeling pressure in her chest. She was having difficulty breathing. It hurt when she took a deep breath and she felt like she wasn't getting enough air. Her leg was also hurting more than it had. Myra took her blood pressure. It was low. Her pulse was fast, she was breathing thirty times a minute instead of the usual twelve to twenty, and she seemed anxious and restless. Myra looked at her lips to see if they were blue, but she couldn't tell because Arlene was wearing thick reddish brown lipstick. She looked at Arlene's nails to see if the nail beds looked blue, but she couldn't see through the sculpted acrylic. She ran to get a pulse oxymeter to measure the amount of oxygen in Arlene's blood. She put it on Arlene's finger and pressed the button. The reading was alarmingly low. Arlene kept repeating breathlessly, "I feel like I'm going to die."

Myra wasn't sure that she was wrong. She picked up the telephone paged Matt Laffey, stat, and called for help.

Seconds later Arlene passed out. By the time everyone got there Myra was trying to force oxygen into her lungs by squeezing a powder blue rubber bag attached to a mask. The code blue team took over. When they hooked her up to an EKG they found that her heart was still behaving. That took some of the urgency away from the moment, but not much. She was still unconscious. Everyone guessed that she had thrown a pulmonary embolus, a blood clot from her leg broke off and went to her lungs. The way it's supposed to work is that you breathe air into your lungs. The air flows down a network of breathing tubes called the bronchial tree. The tubes get smaller and smaller and eventually lead to tiny air sacs. Blood circulates close to the air sacs and the oxygen from the air goes into the blood, which then goes to the heart and finally is pumped throughout the rest of the body through the arteries as oxygen rich blood. When the blood gets to the body tissues, the oxygen leaves and goes into those tissues. The oxygen depleted blood returns via the veins to the lungs for another load of oxygen.

If a blood clot from the leg or somewhere else breaks off and goes into the small vessels in the lungs, it blocks off those vessels. Obviously if the blood can't circulate through the lungs, it can't pick up oxygen. The patient starts breathing rapidly to try to compensate, but sometimes there is just not enough blood getting into the lungs to pick up enough oxygen to sustain the function of the organs. The brain is very, very sensitive to oxygen deprivation.

The other possibility was that they were dealing with a fat embolus. When someone breaks a large bone like the femur, sometimes globules of fat can travel to the lungs and do the same thing as a blood clot. Regardless of the cause, Arlene was sick. She now had much more than a broken leg. They transferred her to the respiratory intensive care unit and called Al Dackel.

By the time he arrived, she was stable but still comatose. Her life was being sustained by a respirator which blew a high concentration of oxygen into her lungs through the plastic tube which had been rammed down her throat in a lifesaving move by a first year anesthesia resident who even amazed herself when she got it in on the first try. Dackel was scared. He knew that many patients in Arlene's condition eventually got well enough to walk out of the hospital, but he also knew that some left from the loading dock. It was too early to tell what would happen to his wife.

He sat by her side and looked at her for a long time without really thinking anything. Then he found himself thinking about their first meeting. It was a blind date arranged by her cousin and his neighbor who themselves had met on a blind date. Arlene was what his father called "quite a looker." Even back then she was extreme, but the times and her youth forgave the excesses. Her hair was a little more teased than everyone else's and her eye make-up was a little heavier, but back then, she was beautiful in his eyes. And in his eyes, today, she was still beautiful.

Arlene had been a very popular girl who always had a boyfriend. Al was pretty much the opposite, but early on, he knew he had to marry her. He asked and she refused. He persisted and she finally accepted. In the early years of their marriage Arlene put all of her energy into making a nice home for her new husband. Everything she did she did for them. But as Al became more and more distracted by his medical training, he became more and more distant and they both became more and more self-absorbed. And for years that was okay for both of them. He had his stuff, she had hers and neither realized, or if they realized they didn't admit, that anything was wrong.

When Brent died, their distance increased. Dackel found more and more things to keep him busy outside of the house and Arlene did the same. All of her excesses seemed to become exaggerated to the point of being almost cartoonish. Dackel suggested counseling but Arlene chose instead to join several women's awareness groups where she spent most of the time talking about what a wonderful life she had.

The next month passed in slow motion. Dackel visited Arlene every day. He saw Capuston a few times. They postponed his deposition. Once, he saw Deborah walking down the street and waved to her, but that was all. He talked to Red, but only when he made the call. From the day of Arlene's accident, Red stopped calling. Dackel was hurt, but he understood that his buddy didn't handle stuff like this too well.

One night, after visiting Arlene, Al got back to his house exhausted and depressed. He opened the door, and heard the usual beeping of his burglar alarm. For the past fifteen years the beeping of the alarm or the ringing of the doorbell or even the sound of a car in the driveway were signals for his Golden Retriever to go nuts. Cookie would drop whatever important assignment she was working on—eating a tissue, lying in the sun, licking herself in a way that humans only wished they could—and she would run to the door. She didn't understand anything about protecting the house or defending her family, she just wanted to see who was there. If she liked you she would jump up and kiss you hello. If not, you might rate a sniff or two before she would go back to her important dog stuff.

For the last year or so, Cookie didn't care much about the doorbell or the alarm. Part of the problem was that she didn't hear so well anymore. That, along with her cataracts, her arthritic hips and some well earned dementia made her a very different dog than she once had been. Her liver was also failing and they didn't expect her to live very much longer. Every time he entered the house Al expected to find her dead. Today the feeling was really strong, and he was relieved to find that he was wrong. She was lying at the foot of his favorite chair in the family room. Without lifting her head she looked up with clouded, tired eyes and, with what looked like more than a little effort, smiled at him as only Goldens can do. She swished her tail only enough to show him that she was glad to see him, and then she closed her eyes and went back to sleep.

She didn't hear the sound of the can opener, but she was still able to smell the Pedigree with Chopped Chicken, her dinner for the last fifteen years. She limped into the kitchen like the old lady she was, but once she was there, she ate like she did when she was a pup, wolfing down her whole supper in seconds and reveling in ecstasy with each gulp.

After she ate he walked her, not as long a walk as in years past, but just enough for her to do her business and sniff around to see who else had done theirs.

When they got back from their walk, Dackel sat in his recliner and made a mental list of all the things that were going wrong: His wife was in a coma; his dog was dying; he was being extorted by a stripper; he was being sued for malpractice; a multimillion dollar corporation was pressuring him to purger himself; he was about to scam an insurance company; his practice was falling apart... His list making was interrupted by the doorbell. Cookie chose to ignore it. Dackel was going to ignore it too, but he didn't. He shuffled over and looked through the peephole. He had no idea who his visitor was but he opened the door anyway.

Bruce Cosmo knew that Dackel had seen his drivers license picture and his private investigator's picture ID, so he used one of his many disguises. He chose one that made him look even scarier than he was in real life. Without introducing himself he simply stated his business.

"Dr. Dackel, I have a business proposition for you."

Dackel realized he never should have opened the door. He was smart enough, however to suppress what would have been his usual arrogant response, or maybe he was just too whipped. He didn't say anything.

"I have in my possession a video tape of you and a young high school girl engaged in various sexual encounters."

Dackel's stomach jumped. His heart raced, but then, in an instant, he calmed down.

"So what," he replied, "I have the same tape."

Cosmo hadn't been sure whether Alice had shown him the tape or not.

"Yes, but has your wife seen it?" asked Cosmo with a sneer.

"Listen asshole, my wife's been in a coma for a month. Look, I told Angel or Carrie or whatever her name is that I'd call the cops if she asked for another nickel, and I'll tell you the same thing. Now get the fuck out of my house."

Sanchez had told him that the guy was a fat wimpy doctor who would cave at the slightest threat. At the moment, that didn't seem so accurate and to further complicate things, Dackel had apparently just trumped one of his aces. He was also somewhat taken aback by the news that Dackel's wife was in a coma. He factored that into his next decision and also considered the wallet thing and that Dackel had refused a reward. He weighed all of those aspects, but business was business. He took a step towards Dackel and put a hand on his right shoulder. He grabbed Dackel's right arm, spun him around and twisted the arm in back of him. He spoke directly into Dackel's ear in almost a whisper.

"The girl won't bother you anymore. It's not money that we want, it's cooperation. We can make this lawsuit go away if you play ball with us. If you don't, we'll give the tape to the tabloids and we'll tell your insurance company about your bogus disability claim. He shoved Dackel into the wall, breaking his nose and loosening at least two teeth. What he didn't count on was that even though he was 58 years old and looked like a marshmallow, Al Dackel was still a South Philly kid who grew up with guys who broke noses and knocked out teeth for fun and made their livings damaging significantly more important organs. He knew how to be tough when he had to be. Besides, he was so depressed about the state of his life that, at that moment, he really didn't care about consequences. He instinctively recovered and threw a roundhouse connecting with the side of Cosmo's head, and knocking him to the floor.

In the movies, this fight would have just been beginning, but in real life, Cosmo was enough of a pro to realize that his job was to deliver a message and nothing more. He got up and got out. And Dackel was reminded, for the first time in about thirty years, exactly how hard the human skull was. When he hit him, his wrist flexed and he felt a searing pain that shot up to his elbow.

Dackel called Red who came right over and took him to the hospital. His nose was broken but they were able to reset it in the E. R. His radius (one of the bones in the arm) was broken and so was a bone in his wrist. After the cast dried, Dackel spoke through his nasal packing, He was angry, but the packing made him sound comical. “You know subthing? The fucki’ guy didi’ eva scare be. I do’t give a fuck if he broadcasts the fucki’ tape on the fucki irnet. He ca’t do aythig about the isurace because we did’t file a claib yet. Ad if he kills be, he kills be. At this poit, I really could’t give two shits.”

Their conversation was interrupted by a nurse who came in to change the packing. When she removed it, there was no further bleeding so she left it out. Dackel signed the discharge papers and he and his friend started walking towards the car.

“Okay, I’ll agree to give up on the disability thing,” conceded Red, “but none of this ‘I want to die’ shit. You’re going through a rough time but you’ve gotten through rough times before and you’ll get through this one.”

“There’s something else, Red,” Dackel said, his eyes filling with tears. He hesitated while he licked his parched lips and swallowed a few times, still tasting blood. Then, he stopped walking, put his hand on Red’s shoulder and turned him so they were face to face. They rarely looked at each other when they talked. He took a deep breath and let out a big sigh, and then he said it. “I don’t miss Arlene. I still love her, but I really don’t miss her.”

Red didn’t know what to say. In the fifty-five years that they had known each other, he and Dackel had never shared a feeling. The best he could do was, “Let’s go home.”

Chapter 26

Dackel hadn't spoken to Deborah in a month. He hadn't been thinking much about his practice and he certainly wasn't in the mood to learn media skills. He did miss her though, but he didn't know that she missed him. She had called a few times but never left a message. He thought of calling a few times but didn't—until tonight. He got her answering machine.

"Deborah, it's Al. Look, I don't think I'm going to be able to continue with your services. Arlene's still in a coma and I broke my arm and I'm really not up for much of anything. Send me a bill for what I owe you and thanks for everything." He hung up and cried.

When he got himself together he left a similar message for Capuston, without the thank you part or the tears.

Dackel's arm was healing well but his wrist was not. It wasn't a typical boxer's fracture. He had broken one of his wrist bones, the navicular, which is the most commonly fractured bone in the wrist. It is also known for not healing well. He tried to remember the "rule of 70's" that he had learned in medical school. He recalled that navicular fractures accounted for 70% of wrist fractures, and that 70% healed well. He couldn't remember the third 70, but he did remember that some patients with navicular fractures went on to develop a condition called avascular necrosis. Basically the bone loses it blood supply and dies. All he knew was that his wrist hurt like hell.

He was unable to do much in the office other than routine examinations and then only with a great deal of pain. His orthopedist told him that he shouldn't be working at all, but his disability didn't kick in for ninety days and so he didn't feel that he could afford three months of no income. More importantly, as it was, he had to send his surgical cases to another doctor and he was concerned that some of them wouldn't come back.

Deborah had called back a few times to see how he was and the last time they spoke, she suggested a locum tenans. These are doctors who are either between jobs, or just like to travel.

Some of them just like to work a few months a year. They come and fill in whenever a situation like this comes up. She knew a reliable agency. Dackel told her to see what she could come up with.

Later that day, Deborah called with good news. A board certified obstetrician gynecologist had just been discharged from the Navy. He planned to start a fellowship in gynecologic oncology in the fall, and he wanted to spend the next six months in Philadelphia to be near his family. He could start in a week. Dackel told her to make the arrangements.

Frank Andrelonis met Dackel in the office at 7 AM. He was a tall good-looking guy with a military haircut. He joined the Navy before college and they paid for his education. He did a residency in obstetrics and gynecology and had been stationed in a variety of exotic and some distinctly non-exotic places. He was now forty years old, single, sober, straight and retired at full pension. He worked hard, by navy standards, and was excited about starting his fellowship. He could have taken six months off, but that wasn't the kind of guy he was. Besides, although he managed to squirrel away a fair amount of money over the years, it was hard to turn down another sixty grand for six months work.

Dackel instantly liked him. He got the sense that Frank was a conservative doctor who was sincerely concerned about his patients. He liked the fact that he was organized and neat. He was impressed with Andrelonis's experience with hysteroscopy and laparoscopy, and his interest in cancer. He hired him on the spot. He just hoped that he could afford to pay him without dipping into his savings, but even if he had to do that, he felt that it would at least keep his practice alive while his wrist healed.

Dackel discovered very quickly that his patients liked Andrelonis too. His only flaw was that he liked to talk and sometimes the office got backed up, but once the patients got in to see him, they felt it was worth the wait. Andrelonis showed Dackel some patient record forms that he had used in the navy. They were organized and easy to work with. Dackel had them duplicated and started to use them. They were precisely the kind of records that QHM required. Andrelonis also instituted a system for following up on Pap smears and mammograms and corrected a billing code in the computer that had probably cost Dackel four or five thousand dollars a year.

Arlene's condition had stabilized. She was still comatose, but the clots were gone and she was breathing with less assistance. The neurologists wouldn't commit to whether or not she would ever wake up, but deep down, they felt that even if she did, she wouldn't have much of a life. She looked like a different person without her makeup and fancy clothes. Her hair had grown out to its normal color, which was one quarter dull brown and three quarters dingy gray. The nurses combed it into two pigtails to keep it out of the way. Some days they would put red ribbons over the rubber bands. The interesting thing was that some who knew her thought she looked prettier now than before the accident. Dackel visited her every day, or at least he stopped by every day. In the beginning he talked to her. He had remembered a neurology professor from medical school who taught that many comatose patients could, at some level, hear. He would put a sign above the bed of every such patient, which read "This person may be able to hear and understand everything you say. Remember to be respectful and careful with your words, and please speak to the patient as if he or she were awake." Although he felt bad about it, and despite his old professor's teaching, he didn't talk to her any more.

Chapter 27

The deposition was held in Sylvan Sheldon's office in a large conference room that doubled as a library. Dackel sat next to his lawyer on one side of the table across from Sheldon and his team. Sheldon liked to bring every available lawyer in his office into his depositions, partly to intimidate the defendant and partly because he wasn't all that bright and he often needed the help. There was one lawyer representing the hospital and three lawyers from a firm representing National Medical Innovations. Paul Shintock was also there. Dackel started to go over to talk to him but Sheldon waved him away. A court stenographer gave a nod and the five-hour torture began.

Sheldon spent a good ten minutes explaining the rules to Dackel, things like, "If you don't hear me, ask me to repeat the question. If you don't understand a question, ask me to clarify. If you need to go to the bathroom, just ask. If you want a drink, let me know."

He then asked detailed questions about Dackel's education. He leaned on every detail. He asked him to name every book he used in medical school, during his residency and since. He asked him to list all of the continuing medical education lectures and courses he had ever attended. He asked what journals he read. Of course, most of the time Dackel couldn't accurately answer him with the detail that he requested. No one could have. This was Sheldon's technique of fatiguing his witness while at the same time pissing him off. Dackel was holding up well. His attorney had coached him and told him what to expect and Metzger-Minkman's media training helped a lot too.

It was close to the end of the second hour when Sheldon started his questioning about Dackel's training in hysteroscopy. Dackel was concerned about this part, but Stacey Finney had told him what to say. He remembered most of it.

"Hysteroscopy, Mr. Sheldon, is a procedure that consists of many components. It requires stabilization of the uterus. I've been doing that several times a day since I started my training almost thirty years ago. Likewise it requires sounding or measuring the uterus which I have done several times a week for the same period. It requires placing an instrument into the uterus which every gynecologist, including myself, can do blindfolded, and it requires looking at a television monitor which speaks for itself."

Sheldon was surprised at the answer. He saw through it, but a jury might not. He needed to recover control of the deposition and try to knock his witness off guard.

"Dr. Dackel," he said squinting and staring Dackel right in the eye, until Dackel turned his head and looked at the clock, "How about the skill required to manipulate the instrument and operate through it? How much experience did you have doing those things prior to Linda Shintock's surgery? How much, Dr. Dackel?" he smirked with adolescent taunting reminiscent of Barry Scheck the diminutive but scrappy DNA lawyer whose fifteen minutes of fame came and went during the O.J. fiasco.

"Objection," shouted Finney, "The procedure never got past the insertion of the instrument. There was no manipulation or hysteroscopic surgery performed in this case."

"But there would have been...," Sheldon snapped back.

"But there wasn't," she said raising her eyebrows high and slowly shaking her head ever so slightly from side to side.

"That has yet to be established, Ms. Finney, and additionally, my experts will testify that there was manipulation performed which indeed led to the injury that ultimately resulted in Linda Shintock's death."

"My objection stands and is noted on the record," snapped back Finney.

"Dr. Dackel, let me explain," she said turning to Dackel. "You may answer Mr. Sheldon's question. I objected because I felt that his question was improper. Since there is no judge here to agree or disagree with me, I put my objection on the record. You answer the question. At some time in the future, a judge will rule on my objection. If he sustains my objection, your answer will be disregarded. If he overrules my objection, your answer will stand. Do you understand?"

Finney knew that Dackel did not need this explanation, but she figured that stopping to explain it to him would interrupt Sheldon's momentum.

"Yes, I understand," he responded.

"Then you may answer the question."

"I forgot the question," he said.

Sheldon, exhaling frustratedly, looked at the stenographer and said, "Please read back the question."

She flipped through several sheets of the narrow paper that had been spewing from her machine and read Sheldon's words in a sing-songy voice that took all the power and acid out of the question, "Dr. Dackel, how about the skill required to manipulate the instrument and operate through it? How much experience did you have doing those things prior to Linda Shintock's surgery? How much, Dr. Dackel?"

Before he could answer, Finney once again stated her objection, for the record.

Dackel hoped he would remember all the things that they had discussed in preparation for this question. He did.

"Mr. Sheldon, I was one of about thirty physicians hand-picked from around the world to learn the operation of the DAC-III. I attended an approved course and received a certificate that states that I successfully completed that course to the satisfaction of the faculty and the university that underwrote the course. I have had as much experience with this instrument as any of the other participants and more than any other gynecologist in the world who was not in attendance."

"That was an impressive answer, Dr. Dackel," said Sheldon." Did you make it up or did Ms. Finney write it down for you?"

"Objection!" said Finney disgustedly, although she had indeed written it for him.

"I'll withdraw that question," said Sheldon, only because he knew that a judge would sustain the objection when the time came. "But you still didn't answer my original question."

"What was the question again?" Dackel asked with his own smirk inside his head that he didn't dare let out.

"Let me rephrase it," Sheldon said. "How much experience do you have with operative hysteroscopy?"

Dackel started to go through his entire rap again starting with "Hysteroscopy, Mr. Sheldon, is a procedure that consists of many components..."

Sheldon was getting frustrated and he started to yell at Dackel, "Just answer the question, Dr., we already saw your dance!"

Under normal circumstances Dackel would have been ballistic by now, but the teachings of his new guru, Swami Metzger-Minkman, taught him to turn the situation into a game. "I'm trying to answer your question, Mr. Sheldon."

Sheldon got control of himself. "Dr. Dackel, had you ever performed a hysteroscopic endometrial ablation prior to the one you performed on Linda Shintock?"

"Objection, he never performed an ablation on Linda Shintock," piped Finney.

"...prior to the one you had planned to perform on Ms. Shintock," he corrected.

"No one outside of the initial research team has performed a DAC-III ablation."

"That's not what I asked, Dr. Dackel," Sheldon said, starting to burn again, "Had you ever performed any kind of endometrial ablation, prior to the one you performed, strike that, planned to perform on Ms. Shintock."

"Objection, irrelevant," said Finney.

"What do you mean irrelevant? How can you say irrelevant? The man was about to do an operation that he wasn't trained to do. How can you say it's irrelevant?" By this time Sheldon was on his feet and pacing. He was waving his arms and shaking his head. He had lost it.

"My objection is noted on the record, Dr. Dackel, you may answer."

"I haven't performed any endometrial ablations prior to planning to perform this one on Linda Shintock, and the reason for that was that I didn't feel that the existing technology was advanced enough to meet my personal criteria for a safe and effective procedure. When I learned the DAC-III ablation technique, and was awarded a certificate of competency after completing the course, I felt comfortable that the operation was safe, effective and that I was qualified to perform it safely and effectively. It was only then that I offered the procedure to Ms. Shintock." He felt bad about lying.

"So this would have been the first endometrial ablation you performed. Is that correct Dr. Dackel?"

"It would have been the first DAC-III ablation performed outside of South America, with the exception of those performed by the researchers in Florida. By the way, did I mention that I was approved by the FDA as a qualified researcher for this device?"

Sheldon ignored his answer. He shuffled through his papers and read notes handed him by his associates. Dackel was getting tired and he felt one of his headaches just starting to let him know that he would be in pain by the end of the day. His wrist was also throbbing. He was hoping no one would ask him about the fluid that he used to distend the uterus. To this point, his testimony was factually accurate, albeit with a practiced spin, but he still hadn't decided what he was going to do if they asked him about the fluid. He hadn't even shared with Finney that he had used plain water during the case.

Even though he was pleased with his performance so far, he felt bad. He saw the combination of sadness and anger in Paul Shintock's eyes, and he kept hearing Linda's last words. He really just wanted to admit to everyone that he had made a terrible mistake and, although it wouldn't even begin to compensate him, write Mr. Shintock a check for the limits of his policy. That's what was going to happen anyway and Paul would have to give 40% plus expenses to Sheldon, the man who gives parasites a bad name. Unfortunately, he was learning that the legal system wasn't especially interested in the truth and, as far as he could see, had nothing at all to do with justice.

"Dr. Dackel, did you hear my question?" Sheldon's voice interrupted his introspecting. "Why did Linda Shintock die?"

"According to the autopsy," answered Dackel, "she died of fluid overload." He wanted to avoid the use of the word water.

"Isn't that another way of saying water intoxication?" asked Sheldon.

"Yes it is," conceded Dackel.

"What causes water intoxication?"

"Objection, don't answer that." interjected Finney.

"What's the problem now?" asked Sheldon.

"He's a defendant. He's not an expert witness."

"But he claims he's an expert hysteroscopist," retorted Sheldon.

"He never made such claims and I instruct him not to answer."

"If he doesn't answer, I'll get a ruling from a judge and bring him back for a continuation of this deposition," threatened Sheldon.

"So be it," said Finney, "Doctor, don't answer the question."

Dackel was very impressed with this kid. She was tough and smart and he couldn't help wondering what his son's life would have been like if he had been allowed to live it.

"Dr. Dackel, according to the statements of some of the operating room personnel, there were cameras in the operating room. Is that true?" asked Sheldon.

"Yes," replied Dackel, once again remembering Finney's instructions to limit his answers to "yes or no" whenever he could.

"And why were those cameras there Dr. Dackel?" He asked in a slow sing-songingly sarcastic manner.

Dackel hated Sheldon but he was not going to allow himself get him angry. "To take pictures counselor."

Everyone smiled including Sheldon's own team. Sheldon didn't smile. Once again, his rhythm was broken. He kept thinking that if this interaction occurred during a jury trial, he would be losing points.

"Take pictures of what?" he asked impatiently.

"Of the whatever they were pointed at." Dackel was getting somewhat carried away, and this answer was even too much for Finney.

"You may answer directly, Dr. Dackel," she said.

"To take pictures of the operation," he said.

"And why would you want to take pictures of the operation? Dr. Dackel?" asked Sheldon.

"First of all," replied Dackel, the FDA requires that the procedure be taped. Secondly, a crew from a television station was taping for a show that they were planning to do, and lastly, so the operation could be broadcast back to National Medical Innovations where they could watch."

"What do you mean 'broadcast back' to National? Why couldn't you just send them a tape?"

On his way to the deposition that morning, Dackel thought long and hard about how he would answer this question. He thought about National's threats and about his wrist. He thought about Linda's last words and the trust that she showed in him. He thought about how he wanted to cancel the case until MacDonald could be there to help, and about the pressure from National and how he didn't want to disappoint Linda. And most importantly, he told himself that whatever he was, he wasn't a liar. But until that moment, wasn't sure how he would answer. When he decided to tell the truth, he felt his soul take a deep breath.

"National's medical director was watching the tape as I was doing the procedure."

"Why was he doing that?" Sheldon asked. Usually he knew the answer to every question he asked during a deposition, but he wasn't really sure that he knew the answer to this one.

"Dr. MacDonald, the medical director had planned to be there but he got snowed out. He was there via Internet to watch the operation and answer any questions I had."

Sheldon's team made a synchronized move for their yellow pads. National's lawyers looked at each other. Sheldon thought that what he had just learned would hurt his case. After all, how many doctors would go to that much trouble to make sure the operation went well. He ended the line of questioning. Had he pushed, Dackel would probably have admitted that he did not feel comfortable doing the procedure alone.

"Ms. Finney, we attempted to get the tape from the television station," said Sheldon, "but they tell us that it had been erased."

"That's true," said Stacey, "we were told the same thing."

"Does National have the tape?" asked Sheldon of the three men in the identical looking blue suits at the far side of the table.

"We'll have to check. We'll let you know," answered two of the three almost in unison.

Jerry Edmonds had instructed his team of lawyers to call him right after the deposition. He was not pleased with what they had to say. It was clear that National was very much involved in the lawsuit.

"Settle it," he told them. "Go as high as two million if you have to."

"That may be tough Jerry, this guy's an asshole and he has delusions of grandeur."

"I said settle it!" He hung up.

The three attorneys from National asked for a meeting with Stacey Finney. They essentially told her that they wanted out and that they would pay whatever it took. She could either join them and make this go away, or finish fighting the case herself and without National's support—or cooperation. Although the last part of the sentence worried her, Finney said that it really wasn't her call. She knew that Dackel wanted to settle, but it was ultimately up to the insurance company.

"I'd also like to see the tape before I make any decisions."

National's lawyers had talked about the tape prior to this meeting and had been assured by Edmonds that it revealed nothing that would demonstrate negligence on National's part.

"We will make an attempt to locate the tape and make it available to you." one of them said. Later, they decided that, for no particular reason, they would wait a few weeks before actually giving it to her.

The tape was delivered to Finney by Federal Express fifteen days later. Sheldon also received a copy. Both attorneys viewed the tape at about the same time, each in his/her office. Neither, of course, had any idea what they were looking at. The left side of the screen showed a calm, orderly operating room. Linda Shintock was smiling up until the moment the anesthesia hit. The tape depicted confident appearing nurses setting up equipment and preparing instruments. It showed a successful test fire of the DAC-III. Dackel even looked like he knew what he was doing. When the hysteroscopy actually started, the picture on the right side of the screen appeared. The lawyers weren't sure what they were seeing, but there was certainly no blood or anything else that looked scary. Then the right side of the screen turned to snow. Missing on the left side was Dimucci tripping. Missing on the right was the flash of light.

Sheldon made a copy of the tape and sent it to his expert, a well respected native Philadelphian who was now Chairman of the Department of Obstetrics and Gynecology at a prestigious medical school in South Carolina.

Finney called Dackel. "I need you to go over this tape with me Dr. Dackel. Can you come this evening after work, like around eight?"

"Sure," said Dackel. His evenings had become very lonely and he was happy to have anything at all to do, and, although he never would have admitted it, he was happy to have an excuse to not visit Arlene. Although she hadn't gotten any worse, she was certainly no better. She was breathing without the respirator, but was still comatose. The last time he spoke to her neurologist, Dackel was told not to be too optimistic. If she recovered at all, it was likely that she would be severely impaired. She did look better though. Dackel found a wig in her closet that Arlene used on bad hair days. He brought it in and asked the nurses to put it on her. As foolish as it seemed, it really made it easier for Dackel to be with her, and he knew that if Arlene was conscious, at any level, she would be grateful.

It was 4:45 and Dackel had three hours to kill. He called Red. They arranged to meet at a small Italian restaurant in South Philadelphia. It was one of those places that seated about twenty five people. They didn't have a non-smoking section, didn't take credit cards and no one ever asked for a menu. You told them what you wanted and they cooked it for you. The one time in forty years that a guy sent something back, he got kicked out and told not to come back.

"So, how's it hangin'?" asked Red.

"Same. Arlene's a vegetable, my wrist hurts like hell, I'm being sued and blackmailed, you know, the usual."

After Cosmo's visit. Red called Jerry Edmonds who swore up and down that he knew nothing about it and it was probably one of Sylvan Sheldon's slimy tricks. Red believed him and advised Dackel to just wait to see what develops.

"What's with this tape thing?" Red asked.

Dackel explained the whole thing but as soon as the veal and peppers came, they stopped talking and ate. When they finished, Red leaned over to Dackel and in an uncharacteristically quiet voice said, "Al, we got to talk about your practice. Your gross is way down, worse than I expected and this new guy is sucking you dry. We gotta do something."

"What the hell am I supposed to do?" fired back Dackel, in a voice much louder than it needed to be.

"I want you to talk to Deborah again. Just talk to her. Maybe we gotta take a different direction with this thing. She knows what she's doing Al, she really knows what she's doing."

"All right. I'll give her a call in the morning."

They paid the check and Red went home. Dackel still had an hour so he just rode around the old neighborhood and thought about the old days.

"What do you mean he turned down two million?" Edmonds was ballistic. "What the hell does he want?"

"His exact words were, 'This case bothers me. I think I can get at least twenty million in punitive damages.'"

"Twenty million? Twenty million? The guy's fucking out of his mind. He'll never get that kind of money!"

"We both know that, but the guy's absolutely crazy. I got the sense that the rest of his firm is relatively reasonable, but it's his name on the door and they kiss his ass."

Edmonds hung up without saying another word. He called Sanchez.

"Get up here now!" he yelled. Sanchez normally didn't like to be told what to do, especially in those tones, but he knew enough to know not to mess with Jerry when he was in one of those moods. He took the stairs, two at a time and was standing in front of Edmonds in less than a minute.

"What's up amigo?"

Edmonds was suddenly very calm. He filled him in. "Pedro, you can't imagine how important it is to this company for this case to go away. If it doesn't, there's a good chance that we'll all be looking for jobs. I don't care what it takes. You have to take care of this. Do whatever you have to."

"Is Sheldon married?" Sanchez asked.

"How the hell should I know?" Edmonds exploded, letting out the frustration and anger that he had, to this point, so nicely contained.

"You know what," Sanchez said, "why don't you leave this to me."

"Fine," said Edmonds, "just fix this and fix it fast!"

Sanchez had his plan formulated by the time he got back to his office. He flipped on his computer and opened up Netscape. He pulled down his bookmark menu and clicked on Switchboard, a web site that could find just about anyone or anything's phone number. He clicked "Business," selected attorneys and typed in Sylvan Sheldon, filled in PA in the "state" box and within five seconds had a telephone number for Sylvan Sheldon Esq. in Philadelphia. He called and asked if Mr. Sheldon was in the office. When he found out he was, he hung up. He then clicked the "People" box and got a phone number in Gladwyne, PA. He dialed the number and got just what he wanted, a maid, probably a Russian.

"Is Mrs. Sheldon there," he asked, hoping that she wasn't.

"No, she is not home now. Can I give a message?"

"Yes," he said, "write this down. Tell her that this is the Marriott Hotel in Philadelphia. Tell her she left her black negligee in the room when she and Mr. Sheldon were here today. We'll mail it to her."

He hung up and looked up the number for a Philadelphia messenger service. He told them he was playing a joke on his friend. He instructed them to go to Victoria's Secret and buy the trashiest black negligee they could find, take off all the tags, spray it with some smelly cheap perfume, take it to the Marriott, ask the front desk for a large envelope, address it to Mrs. Sheldon at the Gladwyn address and mail it from there. He gave them a credit card number and told them to charge him double, and to keep it confidential.

It was an easy little trick that had never failed. She'll get the message. He'll deny that he was in a hotel with anyone. Two days later she'll get the nightgown. Never failed.

Next he walked down to Donny Moline's studio. Donny literally started to sweat when he saw Sanchez. He wasn't sure whether they realized that he had stolen a good deal of equipment over the last few months or that he was using the studio for his personal projects, but he knew that whatever Sanchez wanted, it wasn't good.

"Donny, we got to talk," said Sanchez, "I have a proposition for you. Actually it's for your girlfriend."

Donny was somewhat relieved, but at the same time, he was nervous. How does he know that I have a girlfriend? he asked himself.

"Sure, Mr. Sanchez," he said trying to act relaxed, "what can we do for you?"

"Donny, we know about this Dackel scam you tried to pull. But don't worry, we won't bust you—or kill you, if you help us out."

"Mr. Sanchez, the FBI is already onto us. They told us if we stopped, they wouldn't prosecute and.."

"That wasn't the FBI, it was one of my guys. Sorry. But that's behind us now, isn't it?"

"Yes sir."

"Well this is what we need. Your friend Alice is a good actress and, frankly, quite a piece of ass." Moline knew better than to react. He was right. Sanchez said it to test Donny's self control and his level of fear, both of which were very high at the moment.

"I want Alice to pretend to be a pre-law student and offer to do a volunteer preceptorship in Philadelphia. It will take just a few months and we'll pay her five thousand a month plus expenses. Bring her around tomorrow morning and I'll fill you in."

"I'll see what she says," said Moline.

"Donny, did you hear what I said?" said Sanchez, focusing his eyes right through Moline's, "I said bring her around tomorrow morning and I'll fill you in."

Early the next morning Sanchez was on the phone with Sylvan Sheldon supposedly representing the dean's office at the University of Michigan, Sheldon's almamater, and speaking without showing a single hint of his Hispanic heritage.

"So if you agree, the university preceptorship coordinator will put you on the list. If one of our senior students selects your firm, he or she will volunteer in your office for a semester. This, of course, will not cost your firm anything, and, I'll be honest with you, you'll be getting a bright kid who will work very hard for you. Think about it and get back to me."

"Nothing to think about," said Sheldon, "I'll be happy to host a student."

Dackel was forty minutes early for his meeting with Finney. He sat on a bench outside her building enjoying the breeze and watching the people. He decided that he was going to insist that this case be settled for the limits of his policy. He felt responsible for Linda's death and there was nothing he could do to bring her back. The thing that bothered him most was that he was not even allowed to apologize. Finney told him that if he initiated any contact with Paul or anyone in Linda's family, he would no longer be represented or covered by his insurance company.

Finney led Dackel to a medium sized conference room with a large screen television. She put in the tape and played it for him.

"What do you want to know?" he asked.

"Everything," she replied. "I want to know what was happening at every second of the eleven minutes on both sides of the screen." The left side showed the view of the room as photographed by the news camera. The right showed the picture through the hysteroscope.

"Eleven minutes," Dackel said, "that's how long it took, I worked for twenty five years without losing a patient on the table, and in eleven minutes, just because I was doing something I didn't know how..."

"STOP Dr. Dackel!" interrupted Finney. "Don't say anything, just listen. I've cautioned you before. I just want facts, I don't want commentary."

"I thought lawyers wanted truth," he argued. I want to tell you what happened and I want you to tell Mr. Shintock what happened and I want to settle this case today! I've paid that insurance company sixty eight thousand dollars last year, that's over thirteen hundred dollars a week! They've made tons of money off of me. Now you go tell them to pay up goddammit! It's only fair."

Finney interrupted him. She didn't see the tears starting to pool in the corners of his eyes.

"We've been through this, Dr. Dackel. I told you, that's not how it works. If you want to be your own lawyer, go ahead, but don't expect one penny from your insurance company. Once you start to run this case yourself, you're on your own."

Dackel sighed in despair. "Look, Miss Finney, why don't you let me take the tape home. I'll write a running commentary and I'll bring it back in a few days. I don't really feel like working tonight."

"That's fine with me Doctor, but I'm still going to need to know what happened every second."

"Fine," said Dackel, "I'll call you in a couple of days." He was confused. She wanted to know everything, but every time he started to tell her, she shut him up.

Chapter 28

Alice arrived at Sheldon's office at eight A.M. She decided to use some of the elements of her Carrie Bradford persona, while making sure Dackel wouldn't recognize her, in case they happened to cross paths. She called herself Amanda Mullen from Grand Rapids Michigan. She also made sure she didn't look anything like Angel or Carrie. Alice had the ability to change her entire appearance by changing her hairstyle and her makeup.

"Mr. Sheldon, I can't tell you what an honor it is to work with a man of your stature. I want to be a lawyer more than anything and I can't think of a better way to learn about the field."

Alice worked very hard. One of the first things she did was to steal some of the firm's stationary and mail it to Sanchez as he had instructed. She also sent him a list of the makes and models of all the laser printers in the office. She noted that the standard font used by the word processing department was Courier 12.

By the end of the first week, Alice also picked up some very helpful information. For starters, she heard that Sheldon's wife had walked out on him. Something about an affair that he vehemently denied. He spent much of his time writing her letters and calling her. The feeling around the office was that he was bothered more by the act of her leaving him than the fact that she wasn't there anymore. Sheldon did not like to lose. He had already fired the housekeeper and filed a lawsuit against the Marriott Corporation.

In addition to completing all her of assigned tasks, Alice gathered as much information as she could about the Shintock case. After two weeks, as directed by Sanchez, she started to flirt with Sheldon. If she could get him to her apartment, they would have another tape to work with. If not, she would accuse him of sexual harassment. Whichever, together with the nightgown thing, and one or two other "practical jokes" that Sanchez would orchestrate, Sheldon would be softened up enough to listen to reason. If none of that worked, there was always Plan B.

Alice also learned that it was Sheldon's style not to settle until the last minute, usually not until after the jury was picked. She learned that everyone in the office except Sheldon felt that 1.2 million was a reasonable figure for this case. She learned that there were few other lawyers in the city, and none in his office who had any respect for Sheldon and that he was basically a sad, pathetic asshole. She also found it interesting that she instantly disliked him, even before she knew why.

One of her best wastebasket finds was a "rough draft" of a letter from the expert that Sheldon had hired to review the Shintock case. It really wasn't a rough draft but that's what they called it when they decided that the expert had to make some revisions or clarifications to better support the case. The expert essentially said that he reviewed the hospital records including the operative and the autopsy reports. He also viewed the videotape. It was his opinion, "with a reasonable degree of medical certainty, that although it was probably negligence that resulted in the death of Linda Shintock, there was no evidence of such negligence documented in the material supplied."

There was a sticky note on the letter that read, "If he can't do better than this, destroy this letter and call Parris. Kermit Parris was what is known in legal circles as a "trained seal," an expert who would say whatever the attorney told him to say. There were plenty of them around but Parris was the best, which made him the worst. Because of his reputation as a seal, his nickname was Flipper, even though Flipper was either a dolphin or a porpoise (or maybe they're the same thing). Parris was an eighty year-old retired general practitioner who was never a very good doctor. He reviewed two hundred cases a year and testified in about fifty. He charged twenty five hundred dollars to review a case and five thousand plus expenses to testify.

Sheldon's first choice was to use respected professors as experts, but when he couldn't find one to say what he wanted, he didn't hesitate to bottom feed. He knew that Parris would say whatever he told him to.

Alice faithfully reported to Sanchez every night. Some days there wasn't much to say, but she called anyway. The calls were made to a Philadelphia telephone number that Sanchez had registered in the name of Sylvan Sheldon. The calls were then forwarded by some fancy MCI service to a cellular phone that Sanchez had purchased specifically for this operation. It too was purchased in Sheldon's name. He wanted to be sure that anyone who tried to look into Alice's telephone records would become very confused. He hadn't counted on Alice disobeying his orders and also calling Donny every night.

Dackel put the tape into his VCR and pushed play. He had put this off as long as he could, but Finney kept calling and he knew he would eventually need to look at it. He started to write a narrative, stopping the tape frequently. But every time he started it again, he would lose the first few seconds and have to rewind. It was a pain. He remembered that Deborah had a fancy machine that had all kinds of slow motion and editing functions. Besides he didn't want to watch the tape by himself and mainly, he was also looking for an excuse to see her again, although he would have denied it if you had asked him.

He called her home and Emma answered. "Metzger-Minkman residence, this is Emma," she said in a very professional voice. He really liked the kid. Too bad she was saddled with that stupid hyphenated name.

"Hi Emma, is your mommy home?" he asked in a voice reserved for grandfathers and those who would like to be them.

"Whom may I say is calling?" she replied.

"It's Dr. Dackel, honey," he said.

"My mommy says that men shouldn't call you honey. It's —it's— I forget what it is but you're not supposed to do it."

She's poisoning this child, he thought to himself. Doesn't she ever want her to be normal? But that's not what he said.

"I'm sorry, Emma, I meant to show neither disrespect or chauvinism."

"Nor."

"What?" he asked.

"Nor," she repeated. "Neither disrespect nor showvision and that's the word I couldn't think of."

"You're absolutely right Emma," he said, blushing. He thought about really pissing her off and calling her Emmie, but he decided that he had better things to do than best an eight year old. Instead he just asked to speak to her mommy.

He explained his dilemma to Deborah and asked if he could view the tape at her place. She agreed and they made arrangements for the following evening and then she said something else without even thinking.

"Al, Emma's going to be with her grandma tomorrow, would you like to have dinner first?"

Dackel answered without thinking either. "Sure, how about that Chinese place on Walnut Street at seven?"

"How about The Red Snapper?" she countered, "My treat, I feel like splurging."

"Sure," he said, suddenly feeling very warm in response to what sounded like an invitation to something more than a business meeting.

Sheldon, on the other hand, wasn't responding to Alice's flirting. It seemed to her like it was actually irritating him. She overheard him telling one of his associates that someone was trying to ruin his marriage and she didn't want anyone in the office to suspect her, at least not yet. One night during her telephone update, Sanchez told her to go to the Women's Law Clinic and get them to file a sexual harassment suit. He instructed her to buy a diary and build a good case starting from one week after she started at the firm. She followed his instructions and easily convinced the young, newly graduated and still passionately idealistic lawyer to file a suit.

Once the papers were served, Sanchez knew what he had to do, he just couldn't decide how. Alice knew more than was safe. She was also a professional liar and a documented extortionist. While he was thinking about it, he flipped on the TV and started to watch an old rerun of Cheers. It was the one where someone put a bomb in the refrigerator on Rebecca's rich boyfriend's yacht, and Sam and the rest of them almost got blown up. He remembered how he had laughed the first time he saw that episode. Ever since then he wanted to make a refrigerator bomb.

There were several different ways that he could do this, and he considered many possibilities, but then he remembered once reading about a light bulb bomb. The concept intrigued him. They were relatively easy to make, and left little evidence behind because a light bulb comes with its own initiator and electric ignition system. As he recalled, it was also easy enough to make one in a hotel room with readily available components. He got out his copy of The Terrorist's Handbook and flipped through it until he found section 4.54. He bought a ticket for Philadelphia and made a one-night reservation at the Comfort Inn.

When he got into Philadelphia he rented a car and drove to a K-Mart near the airport. He bought a pack of light bulbs, a butane lighter, epoxy, an Exacto knife, a small box of plastic picnic utensils, a box of plastic bags, six bottles of Snapple and three model rocket kits, gift wrapped. He checked into the hotel and went to work. He placed the light bulb, base up, into a bathroom glass, flicked his BiC and carefully melted the glue that held the glass onto the metal base. He did this very carefully knowing that the inside of a light bulb is a vacuum. When the glue got hot enough, he pulled the metal base off the glass bulb. Once the bulb cooled to room temperature he filled it with rocket fuel. The manual called for black powder or pyrodex, but Sanchez liked rocket fuel better.

Although the typical non-felon might think it was difficult to anonymously obtain rocket fuel, any respectable terrorist knows that model rocket kits came with rocket fuel inside the engines. Basically, the engine is nothing but a heavy cardboard tube surrounding a solid grain of propellant. Sanchez carefully slit the tube with his Exacto and unwrapped it. He removed the gray fire clay from both ends of the grain of propellant with one of the plastic picnic knives. He worked inside a plastic bag so he wouldn't lose any of it if it crumbled. He grasped the grain of rocket fuel with a pair of pliers and ground the pellet until it was the consistency of black powder. The finer he could made it the more surface area would be exposed to the heat. That made for a better explosion. He repeated the operation with the other two kits. After filling the bulb, he glued it back onto the base with epoxy.

He got dressed in a maintenance man's uniform and drove to Sheldon's house. He pulled up on the street in front of the driveway and fiddled with his frequency generator until the automatic garage door opened. It didn't take long for him to find something he could use. An old dusty briefcase that was up on a shelf would do just fine, especially because of the monogram. And oh yes, he left a K-Mart bag with all the leftovers tucked behind a workbench.

He drove over to Alice's apartment and picked the lock in less than twenty seconds. He unplugged the refrigerator, unscrewed the bulb and replaced it with his creation. There were plenty of glass bottles already in there but he added a few more. Each shard of shattered glass would become a potentially lethal projectile once the bulb exploded. He shut the door, and plugged it in again. He left the briefcase, now containing condoms, Astro Glide lubricating jelly and a pornographic bondage video in a closet. In the bathroom he left a few small bottles of shampoo from the Marriott and a Victoria's Secret catalog. Under the mattress he placed a stack of love letters from Sheldon to Amanda typed in Courier 12 on Sheldon's letterhead. Actually they were more like sex letters, but the last included one of those "if I can't have you, nobody will" lines. He was out of the apartment in less than two minutes.

Sanchez was proud of his art and especially pleased with this job. It would take out Alice and ruin Sheldon and no one else would be hurt. He was wrong. The bomb started a fire. The seventy-three year-old building superintendent and her three month-old granddaughter were in the next apartment. They died of smoke asphyxiation, and their deaths hurt a lot of people.

Chapter 29

Dackel had never been to the Red Snapper. It was supposed to be one of Philadelphia's most elegant restaurants. He knew he was not elegant. He didn't hang with elegant people and he didn't like it when every time he shifted position, a waiter of questionable sexual orientation adjusted his napkin, which happened to him once at an upscale restaurant in San Francisco.

He pulled up in front of the restaurant and gave his keys to the valet. When he heard it cost ten dollars to park, he grabbed the keys back and drove around until he found a space. It was a little close to a fire hydrant, but he parked there anyway.

Deborah was sitting at the bar when he got there. Dackel was surprised at how pretty she looked. Even her overbite was kind of cute. She was wearing a long black v-neck dress that was very flattering to her bust line, she had on normal shoes, and she was wearing makeup. Dackel wore a white turtleneck that was not at all slimming, and a muddy green jacket. Had she been conscious, Arlene would have never let him out of the house with that outfit, but, then again, had she been conscious, he would have never been at the Red Snapper with Deborah Metzger-Minkman.

"This is not a date," was the first thing he said when he saw her. "I'm still married and this is a business meeting." Shortly thereafter he told her that she looked very pretty. They were seated towards the back of the restaurant as if the hostess instinctively knew that, at some point during their dinner, there would be some sort of embarrassment coming from their table. She wasn't disappointed.

Dackel complained that it was too dark and that he couldn't understand most of the menu. He spilled his wine twice. His most Dackelesque move, however, was whistling for the waiter when he wanted more bread. Metzger-Minkman didn't seem to mind his behavior. Although not nearly as crass, she was like Dackel in a lot of ways. She was an educated woman. (He was educated too.) She was good at what she did. (So was he, as long as he limited himself to what he could do.) She was unpolished in certain areas. (He was unpolished in most.)

At first it was awkward. They would both start to speak at the same time and then both would stop to let the other continue. Once they settled down they spent most of the next two hours learning about each other. She told him that she too grew up in South Philadelphia. She worked her way through Temple University night school. While she was in school she worked as a secretary for a hot shot medical practice consultant whom she eventually married. He was shot in the head by a fourteen year old who robbed him of twenty dollars at an ATM machine two blocks from their home.

He grew up just as poor. He told her about pharmacy school, including why he got kicked out, how he took a shot at med school and got in, and how his son died. He told her how he met Arlene on a blind date at the World's Fair in New York and how when he went to meet her folks in their Brooklyn apartment, how rich he suddenly felt living in a row house. He told her that he didn't expect Arlene to ever come home.

They both shared more than either of them usually shared and Dackel did something he never did. He took a forkful of his refried risotto and offered it to Deborah. She accepted and allowed him to feed it to her.

They sat there long after they finished dinner. There was another party waiting for their table but despite all the waiters tricks, they just sat there. He didn't realize that he was falling in love. All he knew was that he was connecting with someone in a way that he never knew existed. At this point all she acknowledged was that he was a decent guy who was catching all the red lights of life, and that she felt sorry for him. At one point she did reach over and brush a crumb from his chin with the corner of her napkin. She didn't realize that those who studied body language would consider that courting behavior.

The waiter brought the check. The busboy cleared the table. Al and Deborah continued to talk. They took the linen off of the table. The conversation continued. Finally the hostess just came right out and told them that someone was waiting for their table. She apologized profusely. He shrugged his shoulders.

They walked back to Deborah's office and put in the tape.

"We'll watch it through once, then we'll go back and do stop action while you dictate what's happening. My secretary can transcribe it in the morning," suggested Deborah. He hadn't thought about dictating his narrative.

"That a great idea," he said touching her on the shoulder. Other than a handshake early on in their relationship, that was the first time he ever touched her. His penis didn't twitch, but he did feel a chill start at his shoulders and ripple through his body. She, on the other hand, experienced the female equivalent of a twitch. That's where it ended, at least for that night. They both pulled back and started to watch the tape. When it was over, her brow was as wrinkled as a basset hound's.

"Something's very strange here," she said slowly. "Where's the flash of light and the kid tripping?"

"Maybe the camera didn't get the kid, and what flash of light are you talking about?"

Deborah went to the bottom drawer of a filing cabinet and took out the two tapes that she had gotten from her friend at the TV station. One was what the camera crew shot and the other was the view through the hysteroscope. They had been fed together on one screen to MacDonald. She hadn't really intended to save them, so she put them in with the blanks and figured she'd use them to record E.R. or Sixty Minutes. She put one in the VCR and pushed play. The beginning was the same, but then you could clearly see Dimucci trip and fall against the DAC. There was a time code on the bottom of the tape. It looked like a digital stopwatch recording the number of hundredths of a second the tape had been running. Video editors used time code to synchronize two tapes shot at the same time.

"Okay, he trips at about six minutes and ten one hundredths of a second. Now hand me the hysteroscope tape."

She played the tape and at six minutes and ninety-three one hundredths of a second there was a flash of light on the screen, and then the blood. Dackel explained that the monitor had quit at that time, but the camera and tape recorder were still working. The tape that they were looking at should have been a combination of these two. It clearly was not.

"This tape has been edited Al. Where did it come from?"

"As far as I know, from National Medical Innovations."

"Al, we have to call your lawyer. This is evidence and it's been tampered with. If they find out, they may accuse you."

"Accuse me? I can't even get my goddamn VCR to stop blinking 12:00, how are they going to accuse me?"

"Trust me Al, We can prove by the time codes that this tape has been altered. I'll help you but you have to call your lawyer first thing tomorrow."

It was after midnight. Any romantic hormone surges that might have been there earlier in the evening had been replaced by adrenaline in her and nausea in him.

When Dackel got back to his car he found the drivers side window smashed in. His radio and car phone were gone and there was a cat sitting on his dashboard. He also found a twenty five dollar ticket on his windshield.

Chapter 30

At first, the fire department assumed it was a gas stove explosion. The stove in Alice's apartment did, in fact, blow up, but the arson investigator knew better. Although he didn't figure out that it was a light bulb bomb, he knew that the charge was somewhere in the back of the refrigerator. He also found the suitcase and the letters. What they were not able to find was the identity of the young woman who had been burned, dismembered and disemboweled beyond recognition by thousands of glass missiles. They could find no record of an Amanda Mullen from Grand Rapids. The University of Michigan had no Amanda Mullen registered nor did they have a preceptorship coordinator.

The police questioned Sheldon for four and a half-hours. He denied writing the letters and he denied having an affair with Mullen. But he was the kind of lawyer who never thought twice about lying and just about every one in Philadelphia knew it. Now that he was finally being honest, no one believed him. It was a twist on the old fable which could now be called, "The Boy Who Cried Truth."

Donny hadn't gotten his nightly call for over a week. When he dialed Alice's Philadelphia number a recording said the number was no longer in service. When he called Sheldon's office, all he was told was that she hadn't been in all week. Sanchez told him that she just disappeared. Donny was more pissed than worried. He loved Alice, but he knew she was a hustler and a free spirit and he expected that someday she would just take off if her money divining instinct or any of her less unique senses were tempted. He didn't even consider the possibility of foul play. He also didn't realize that he was next.

Sanchez decided to kill Donny with carbon monoxide. His plan would also allow him to try something he had been meaning to play with for a long time. It was called the "date rape drug," but from what Sanchez understood, it would suit his needs very well. The proper name was Rohypnol, but on the street they were known as "Roofies", "Ruffies", "roche", "R-2", "rib" or "rope."

Rohypnol is nothing more than a tranquilizer similar in nature to Valium but much more potent. It works in about a half-hour to produce a sedative effect, and muscle relaxation, but it also causes amnesia. Sanchez first learned about Rohypnol in the late 1970's, but it didn't hit the streets of Tampa until the early 90's. It was usually slipped into someone's drink, and after about a half-hour the slipper could do pretty much whatever he wanted to the slippee. On college campuses, it was usually the woman who was given the drug and then raped. In bars, it was occasionally a woman who picked up an affluent looking man, took him back to his place, dropped a roofie in his martini and then left with his money and jewelry.

He knew he could have had some sent by one of his contacts in Mexico where it is available over the counter in any farmacia, but instead, he went to a bar a mile from his office and bought ten of them for twenty bucks.

Sanchez called Donny on the pretense of wanting to talk about Alice and where she might be. He met him at a nostalgia burger place near the office, dropped three pills in his milkshake and waited. Before long, Donny's speech began to slur, and he started to drop his fork. His eyes started to look bloodshot.

"You're looking sick," said Pedro, let me drive you home in your van. I'll take a taxi back here to pick mine up."

He drove Donny back to his apartment and pulled into an empty corner of the parking lot and put Donny, now comatose, in the driver's seat. He left a note on the dashboard, typed of course, and used a basic "hose in the tailpipe" technique. When he was sure no one was looking, he got out of the van and walked for about three miles. He took a bus back to the restaurant and picked up his car.

What Pedro didn't count on was that Donny was a long time pill-head and he had built up an incredible tolerance to the class of drugs called benzodiazepines, one of which was Rohypnol. He woke up before the carbon monoxide hit and was able, barely, to open the door and fall out of the van. He didn't fully come out of it for another two hours. When he did, he saw the hose and the note. Even through his stupor, he knew what was happening. His van was out of gas so he staggered to the road and hailed a cab to the airport. He bought a one way ticket to Philadelphia. He would stop by Alice's apartment and see if anyone knew where she was. Also, Barry Wilson, a guy he used to work with, lived in Philadelphia and he was sure he could crash there for a while.

Chapter 31

Dackel dialed Stacey Finney's number at exactly 9 A.M. and braced himself for the all time world's speed record telephone greeting "DaggetLaurelStrattonBinsley&Rittenhousecanyouhold," followed by at least four minutes of smooth jazz. When the receptionist came back on, he asked for Stacey. Of course she wasn't there. She never was. He left an urgent message and went back to work, and judging from his list of patients, he realized it would indeed be work. Glancing down the schedule he saw a test demander, a test refuser and a test distruster.

The test demander usually came in with a ream of magazine pages torn from the medical journals of the masses (Glamour, Ladies Home Journal, Prevention and the like.) She would always ask for every test available. Once, this particular one demanded an amniocentesis to check for Down's syndrome. It took several minutes to convince her that the test was only for pregnant women and that a 64 year-old really didn't need it.

The test refuser felt in her heart of hearts that tests caused the diseases that they checked for. She had known women who had annual mammograms and then developed breast cancer, and an uncle of hers who was a miner got lung cancer. She was sure it from the x-rays. Even the Pap smear was dangerous in her mind.

Some of his most eccentric patients were test distrusters. This particular distruster always requested that her mammography be read by a minimum of three different radiologists and she requested that at least one of them be Jewish. She herself was not Jewish, but she felt that Jewish doctors were more careful because they were more afraid of being sued.

The funny thing was that each of these patients had some valid points. It wasn't unusual for something to show up in a test that a patient requested, and there is no doubt that some tests do have risks and complications associated with them. It also makes sense that the more eyes that look at an x-ray, the greater the likelihood of making an accurate diagnosis.

As he was about to see his first patient, Stacey Finney returned his call. Dackel filled her in about the tape. She asked that he bring it to her immediately. She would have the tapes analyzed and compared by a video technician who had testified for her before. He was supposedly the best in the city. His name was Barry Wilson.

Dackel told her that he was in the middle of office hours and he couldn't possibly get over to her office before five. Totally out of character, Finney told him to have it ready for her, and she would pick it up in a half-hour.

Stacey Finney was at Dackel's office twenty minutes later and twenty minutes after that she was at Barry Wilson's door. Usually she would have had it delivered by messenger, but she wasn't trusting anyone these days. Besides, she had a two-hour hole in her schedule she could now charge to Dackel's insurance company. When she joined the firm she was advised by one of the partners to try to bill at least eleven hours for every eight that she worked.

Barry had a state of the art studio and knock-your-socks-off apartment in a loft which used to be part of a cigar factory. You could still faintly smell the aromatic tobacco which had become one with the walls. Barry had the latest digital equipment, an incredibly souped-up Macintosh and the skill to make him the best in the business. He was as good at altering tapes as he was detecting alterations. Dagget Laurel had used him for both. He was expensive but worth it. He was also one of the new generation of nerds who, by virtue of their brains and money, achieved instant stud status. Stacey had been in his power and his bed more than a few times. That was another reason she took the tape over herself.

Barry was out on a job. She left the tape with a friend who was visiting. She had no way of knowing that this was not the first time Donny Moline had handled those tapes. He didn't make a very good impression that day either. He needed a shave and he looked as if he had a hangover. She thought about waiting for Barry, but Donny kind of scared her and, anyway, with him there, it wasn't likely that she would have the opportunity for an early afternoon delight. She gave Donny the manila envelope with the two tapes, and stopped into the bathroom, to take her panties out of her briefcase and put them back on. She went back to her office, disappointed, and with a residual arousal which frustratingly lasted for the rest of the day.

When Barry got back he read the note that she left with the tapes and put them into two side by side decks. Moline was napping. Although it was supposedly physiologically impossible for the eye and the brain to do, a good video technician was able to see a tape almost frame by frame. A few seconds after the first edit, he started to laugh out loud. He knew instantly that the tape from National had been altered. He also knew that it was done by someone almost as good as he was. Of course, he also knew who that was.

"Hey asshole, wake up," he said trying to control his laughter. "Look at this."

Donny was somewhat out of it, but he was awake enough to see what was going on.

"Where did they possibly get the original?" he asked. Barry told him that according to the letter, it had been supplied by the Defendant's media consultant. Donny pushed stop and told Barry to make himself comfortable. He told him the whole story starting with the first time he met Alice in a massage parlor and finishing with his latest brush with the ultimate erase head.

"The question is what to do now," he said.

"Okay, lets look at the options," replied Barry, always the one to logically lay out the alternatives and then, without emotion, fear or ethical consideration, pick the option best for him. "Obviously they are going to find out the tape was altered and obviously it's going to come back to you. But what did you do? You edited a tape. Your boss told you to clean it up and you cleaned it up. They just might have wanted it cleaned up for instructional purposes. You didn't know anything about a lawsuit. So, you could play dumb. But, if they somehow link you and Alice, and find out that Alice was spying, that could complicate things. Is she the kind of girl who'd rat you out? If you trust her, I think you ought to tell Stacey that you edited the tapes and tell the cops that someone tried to kill you. These guys are going down and you want to be as far away from them as you can be."

"I don't know," Donny said, "these guys don't mess around. I'm afraid of them, and I really don't know how much I trust Alice."

"Look buddy," said Barry, "if they find you, and they will, you're toast. You know way too much. I don't see what you have to lose, but let's run it by Stacey. I can trust her, as much as you can trust any of them."

"Any of what?" asked Donny, "lawyers or women?"

"Yeah," answered Barry, with a snicker.

"Maybe," said Donny, "but I need to think about it for a while. I'm going to walk over to Alice's apartment and see if the super knows where she went. How do I get to the Fairstone Apartments."

Barry froze. "The Fairstone?"

"Yeah, it's somewhere around here, isn't it."

Barry walked over to Donny and guided him to a chair.

"Man, I don't know how to say this, so I'm just going to say it. There was an explosion at the Fairstone and an unidentified woman in her twenties was killed."

Donny ran to the bathroom and threw up everything there was to throw. His decision was made.

Stacey Finney hung up the telephone. Barry Wilson told her that the tape had been altered and by whom. He told her about the attempt on Donny's life and he told her that he was pretty sure of the identity of the bomb victim and the bomber and the links between Alice and Sheldon and Alice and National. It was a long conversation and she took a lot of notes. Once she sorted it out she called a meeting of all of her senior partners, something that young associates just don't do, but there was an urgency and an authority in her voice that made the managing partner curious.

"Tell me what you have," said Jerome Binsley. She did. He got on the phone and called a meeting for three that afternoon.

The partners were all in their chairs by 3:35. Binsley did something that was unheard of. He gave the floor to Finney. For the next forty minutes she presented her case in an organized and compelling manner. She referred to her notes only a few times and took only one sip of water, which she did more for dramatic effect than from thirst. When she finished they knew a few things. They knew they were going to have to give her a raise. She would ask before the end of the day. They also knew that they had an ethical dilemma. They had information that would get Sheldon off the hook for Alice's murder. They knew they would have to notify the authorities, but they didn't want to just give it away.

"How do you think we should go with this, Ms. Finney?"

She hadn't really had the time to think that out. She assumed that they would decide as a group. She also would not have been surprised if they took the case from her.

"This is the first case I've ever had with Sylvan Sheldon, but my initial impression is that he's crazy. What I would do is, how should I say this, attempt to settle the Dackel matter before we release this information. We might hint that we have information that..."

"That will be enough, Ms. Finney. I don't think it would be a good idea for anyone to hear any more. You will remain on this case and attempt to settle it as quickly as possible according to your client's wishes. I will deal with the insurance company. You can—negotiate with Mr. Sheldon."

Every one of the partners knew exactly what was going on. Finney would use the information as a way of extorting a reasonable settlement. If it went bad, they would deny knowledge of her tactics and fire her ass.

Chapter 32

Arlene was doing pretty much the same. The last time Dackel spoke to the neurologist, and that was more than a week ago, they decided that it was time to try to find a long term care facility. It was not likely that Arlene would ever wake up. The nurses had long abandoned the wig and the fancy nightgowns. Arlene was gray and thin and old. Her muscles had long since wasted and if you touched the loose wrinkly skin of her thigh, a thigh from which Dackel had once, albeit long ago, derived sexual pleasure, it felt as if the flesh could be pulled right off of her bone.

The social worker helped him find an extended care facility in Bucks County, about forty minutes from Philadelphia. It was expensive and it was unlikely that her insurance would pay very much of the cost. But he signed the papers and she was transferred. Dackel sat by her bedside and talked to her while they waited for the transfer ambulance. He hadn't spoken to her for a while and frankly, he didn't really think she could hear him today. He didn't realize it, but he was really talking to himself.

"Arlene, I've learned a lot about myself in the last few months. I realize that I haven't been the best husband in the world, emotionally, that is. You know, I didn't really know how to share my feelings. I just never learned how. And I guess I didn't communicate as well as I could have. Who knows what our marriage would have been like if I had. You might have even given me a blow job, heh heh" he chuckled. "But seriously, we did pretty good together and I'm sorry you can't see that I have changed a little bit."

He stopped talking and just thought the rest of what he wanted to say, just in case she was able to hear him.

"Arlene, I've never been one to gush all over you and tell you I love you ten times a day." Actually he probably hadn't told her he loved her ten times in their marriage. "But I guess I do. I gotta be honest. There wasn't much passion the last few years. We were both too busy, I guess..."

He couldn't even silently say what he wanted to say next, that he was sorry she was in a coma but he wasn't sorry she was not actively involved in his life any more. He couldn't say, even to himself, that Deborah showed him a new side of himself and that he thought he was in love with her. He couldn't even begin to admit that he was ready for Arlene to die. He started to speak out loud again.

"So - uh I don't really know what I wanted to say so I guess I'll say good-bye for now." What he really wanted to say was good-bye —period. Oh, he would visit her every week, but emotionally, he had said good-bye. It was interesting that Arlene's friends didn't even say good-bye. They just stopped visiting after a month or so. Her only family, her sister visited every week, but only for a few minutes. She spent most of the time complaining about the heat in the room and the smell and just about everything else.

Chapter 33

At Deborah's suggestion, Dackel asked for another meeting with QHM. As much as he hated the HMO, he really needed them. He brought with him the new medical record forms he was using, and he acted very humble (Deborah helped him practice.) He told them about his wife's illness and his wrist and about Andrelonis. He asked what he could do to convince them to allow him back in. They said they would get back to him. They never did. He wanted to discuss the problem with Andrelonis but he didn't know how to tell him that he couldn't afford him.

Andrelonis beat him to the punch. The next day there was a yellow sticky note on his desk. It said, "Boss, save some time for me today, I'd like to talk to you."

"Shit," thought Dackel, "I bet he's going to quit." He went through the day in a bad mood trying to figure out what he was going to do. His wrist was no better and he hadn't been able to work very much, but he still came into the office a few days a week. He also liked the idea of having Andrelonis do the surgery. He even began recommending *alterrrnative* surgery to appropriate patients. He also liked having someone else to talk to about tough cases, and he liked it when Frank asked him for his opinion. He really didn't want to see him go, but then again, he couldn't afford to keep him.

Frank got back from the operating room close to five o'clock. He smelled from a combination of sweat and rubber gloves, and he had a thin red dent just below his hairline from the elastic O.R. cap.

"How'd it go?" asked Dackel.

"The first case went fine, but I had some trouble getting the dermoid out through the laparoscope."

A dermoid, or more officially, a benign cystic teratoma, is one of the strangest tumors in medicine. Dermoids account for about one out of every six or seven ovarian tumors. As their name indicates, they are usually benign. They come from the cells that usually make the eggs. If the egg is fertilized by a sperm, a baby develops, but every once in a while, for reasons no one knows and without the benefit of fertilization, one of the egg producing cells starts to develop in an unstructured, chaotic manner creating a dermoid. These weird tumors contain clumps of hair, pieces of bone, globs of fat and sometimes fully formed teeth. Dackel always made an incision to remove them. Andrelonis usually took them out using laparoscopic or belly button surgery techniques.

"So," said Dackel nervously, "what do you want to talk to me about?"

"Al, I want to buy into your practice. I like your patients, I like your philosophy, I like working here. I decided that I don't want to do the fellowship."

Al was shocked. He was relieved, but he was shocked. After the poison that his last associate spit before she left, he was convinced that no one would ever want to work with him, let alone pay him money to join him.

"Frank, as far as I'm concerned, you're in," said Dackel grabbing Andrelonis's hand and pumping it like he was jacking up a car. "We'll get the accountants to figure the deal, but whatever it is, you're in."

For the moment, Dackel was happy. Jerry Edmonds was not. He heard the bad news from a friend of his who worked for a very well known medical equipment manufacturer. Three of their top executives had been fined eighteen million dollars each conspiring to hide potentially deadly flaws in medical equipment. The company was fined sixty one million.

"We must settle the Shintock case," he told his lead attorney. "Go talk to Sheldon again. From what I understand, he's taken a few weeks off but I think you'll be able to find him. Offer him five million with a confidentiality clause."

"Jerry, I don't think that a jury would fault us for the death. The machine wasn't the problem, it was..."

"I don't give a fuck whose fault it was, I want this case settled and I want it settled quietly. No—make that silently."

"Whatever you say, Jerry, but you're going to have to answer to the board."

"Let me handle the board. You go find Sheldon," screamed Edmonds.

Sheldon's secretary called him at home. Stacey Finney told his secretary that she needed to talk to him urgently. His response, through his secretary, was that they had nothing to talk about. Finney's retort was that she was happy to respect his wishes, and she would be happy to wait until he got situated in prison. If, however, he could possibly find a few minutes for her now, he might not have to go. When his secretary relayed that message, he granted her an audience. They met in her office an hour later.

"Sylvan, let me tell you a few things. Number one, I think you have no ethics. Number two, your ego is sucking the life out of your common sense."

"That's enough you young little hot shot. I was around before..."

"Please, Sylvan," she cut him off, "let me finish. Number three, you have delusions of grandeur about this case. And numbers four and five, I know you didn't kill the girl and I know who did."

"What? Who? Tell me..." he stammered.

"Just keep listening. I'm going to tell you about a hypothetical deal, and that's just what it is, nothing more. If you think it's a good hypothetical deal, tell me so, if you don't, this conversation never happened. I want you to suppose that a defense attorney would propose to a plaintiff's attorney such as yourself, who was representing a client such as Mr. Shintock to take eight hundred thousand to settle a case similar to Linda Shintock's.

Suppose, hypothetically, of course, the operating surgeon in that case had great remorse about the incident, but felt that it was as much the company's fault as it was his. Suppose he has signed a 'consent to settle' and the carrier had agreed to the aforementioned number. I'd also like you to suppose that the terms of this settlement call for the plaintiff's attorney to drop the punitive damages from his case and further suppose that the terms of the settlement will be kept strictly confidential. Suppose that the agreement called for a document stating that if the plaintiff's attorney leaked any of the terms of the agreement, he would forfeit his percentage of the settlement to the defendant doctor.

Suppose again that the agreement allowed the plaintiff's attorney to pursue his case with the equipment manufacturer and the hospital, but suppose that if he does, he may not mention the defendant doctor's name nor call him as a witness, and in the event that he is called to testify by the other defendants, he will not be cross examined. Finally, suppose that in exchange for this settlement, information will be provided which will most assuredly clear the name of the plaintiff's attorney with regard to any current criminal investigation."

"God damn it Stacey, cut the legal talk and the blackmail and tell me what you know!"

"Did I say I knew anything?"

"Hey, this is my ass, I've been framed and if you had anything to do with it, I'll personally see to it that..."

"Slow down Sylvan, you heard my hypothetical, what do you think?"

"This is highly unprofessional, Stacey. You are trying to extort me. I could have you disbarred for this shit."

"I just want you to think about a reasonable settlement," Stacey said calmly.

"But I don't know what I'm dealing for. Tell me what you know and I'll think about it," said Sheldon regaining his professional negotiation posture.

"This meeting never happened," Finney said as she got up and opened the door.

He sat there for a moment. Had this been any other negotiation, he would have walked. He knew that when someone approached him with a settlement offer, he usually had the upper hand, but this was different. It was his ass, and no client was more important than that.

"Okay, you got a deal," he conceded. "Tell me what you know."

Finney reached into her briefcase and pulled out a three page agreement which Sheldon scanned and quickly signed. Of course, just in case he didn't sign his name, he just scribbled the words, "Do not Agree." Stacey didn't bother to examine the signature. She told him what she knew about the tape, about Moline and Alice and MacDonald and about what really happened that day in the operating room. She didn't tell him about the sterile water that Dackel mistakenly used because she didn't know about it. At this point the only one who did was Dackel.

"We still don't know why she died, do we?" Sheldon asked.

"No, we don't," she answered, "and we may never know. But I do know that National should never have left him alone with the machine and I know that they know it too. As I see it, the attorney general and the FDA both need to know about this case and so do the Philadelphia and Tampa police departments."

"What I have to decide," he said slowly regaining his plaintiff's attorney demeanor, "is how I want to play it with them. But I'll work that out. In the meantime, give me the papers back."

"Why?" she asked.

He reached across the table and snatched the papers from her hand and in a move very unlike Sylvan Sheldon, he resigned the agreement with his real signature. When Stacey realized what he had originally signed, she blushed a deeper red than anyone had ever blushed before.

"I guess I'm not as smart as I thought," she said sheepishly.

"You're plenty smart and you got balls," Sheldon answered, "and anytime you want to make some real money, you got a job with me."

Finney felt, at that moment, just like she did when she was asked to the prom by the fat kid with the Thomas's English Muffin (with strawberry jelly) complexion and the ear wax that was visible from thirty feet away.

"Thank you, I'll keep that in mind," she said, struggling to hold back her lunch.

At about that time, National's lead attorney was on the phone with Sheldon's secretary.

"Please give Mr. Sheldon the message that we have an offer for him that is consistent with his demand," were the words they used. They knew they weren't going to give him 20 million, but they knew when they handed him a check for five, he wouldn't be able to turn it down. When Sheldon got the message he responded quickly and surprisingly calmly.

"Yeah, well I have an offer for you," he said when he returned the call. "I'll be there in the morning."

Stacey Finney called Dackel at home but he wasn't there. From the number of beeps on his answering machine, it sounded like he hadn't been there for a while. He hadn't. He had been to the mall. This was a new experience for Dackel. Before he got married, his mother bought all of his clothes, even his shoes. Then Arlene took over. But he needed underwear. He didn't even know his size. He had to look at the label. Hanes 42's he wrote on a small piece of paper and headed off to the mall.

At first he was overwhelmed. Bloomingdales, Sears, Penny's, he didn't know where to start. Fortunately, he quickly found what he needed. After he bought them he walked to the door, but discovered that it was pouring and his car was at the other end of the world. He went back in and sat on a bench and did something else that was new for him. He people-watched. He looked at the different sizes and shapes of people. He watched them interact. He tried to guess what they were thinking. It all felt so strange to him, but it relaxed him and he liked it. The rain stopped, but he stayed. He stayed until closing time.

When Dackel got home there were five messages. Arlene's doctor called. She had a kidney infection that wasn't clearing up and they wanted permission to consult with an infectious disease specialist and a urologist. Deborah called, just to see how he was doing. Red called to tell him that 9 1/2 weeks was on Showtime, and MCI called for the usual annoying reason. The final call was from Stacey Finney. After the beep he heard what sounded like an excited teenager.

"Dr. Dackel, good news! We settled your part of the case. I'll call you with the details tomorrow.

Dackel let out a deep breath. His visit to the mall had mellowed him out, and despite all the things that were wrong in his life, he started to feel more calm, serene and even optimistic. He liked the new thoughts and feelings he was allowing himself to have, and he actually liked the person he was becoming. He felt very relieved that the case was over.

But an hour later he wasn't feeling so great. Something was wrong. With the news of the settlement, he expected that a big weight had been lifted from his chest, but he was starting to feel just the opposite. He felt a pressure building, like someone was sitting on his chest. The back of his neck was also feeling tight and his left arm was sore. He also felt starved for breath and he was nauseated and sweating profusely. He knew what was happening. He took an aspirin, dialed 911 and then passed out.

Dackel didn't remember fire rescue breaking down his door and transporting him to the hospital. Fortunately, he didn't need CPR and he was stable and awake by the time he was transferred to the cardiac intensive care unit. It was not an impressive unit. There were four beds staffed by two nurses and a relatively green intern. When he found out that Dackel was a doctor, he called his attending staff who didn't seem to care all that much.

The next morning it was confirmed that he indeed did have a heart attack, and a pretty decent one. Everyone agreed that he should be transferred to Fourteenth Street Hospital for further evaluation. He asked that the nurses notify Deborah, Red and Andrelonis. They never got around to it.

He was feeling somewhat better and his pain was gone, but he felt exhausted by the time he arrived at Fourteenth Street, and he was scared. He was taken immediately up to the coronary ICU and scheduled later that day for a cardiac catheterization. The cardiology fellow told him that the aspirin may have been what saved his life by making his blood less sticky. Dackel had fortunately remembered a study that he just happened to see that showed that a single aspirin taken at the time of a heart attack did something good. He hadn't remembered what, but he had the presence of mind to take one.

He watched the door for Deborah or Red or someone, but no one came. There were no bedside phones in the ICU so he asked his nurse to call Deborah again. She did better than that. She brought a phone over to him and he dialed.

"Hello, you have reached Practice Doctors. We aren't available at the moment, but your call is very important to us. Please leave a message after..."

He tried to leave a message that wouldn't alarm her, but he broke down crying in the middle. The nurse took the phone and left a number. She sedated Dackel and he slept until they woke him for his cardiac catheterization.

He had never seen an actual cardiac cath, but he knew what to expect. They put him on a special table, prepped his groin with Betadine, the way he had prepped many groins over the years, and gave him an injection of local anesthesia. Whenever he injected local, he always told his patients that, "this is going to feel like a little bee sting." After this, he would leave out the "little" part.

T. Russ Hayman, the interventional cardiologist then pushed a needle into a large blood vessel in Dackel's groin and passed a plastic tube through the needle. The tube or catheter snaked its way up to his heart. When it got to the right spot, the doctor injected some dye and started to take x-rays. Everyone in the room watched the television monitor as the dye filled the arteries that nourish the heart muscle. Everyone also saw the problem. The left anterior descending artery narrowed suddenly. That corresponded to the area of heart damage that showed up on the electrocardiogram.

"It looks like one vessel," said the tech who was assisting.

"Yep," said Russ. Get me my balloons."

The tech handed Russ another long catheter. He carefully passed it up to the area of obstruction and gently nudged it through. Once it was in position he pushed the plunger of a syringe, which inflated a balloon that he had positioned just inside the narrowed artery. As the balloon inflated, the artery widened and blood started to flow through. What was actually happening was that the plaque that had accumulated in the wall of the artery was being cracked and the artery was allowed to expand. Hayman then inserted another catheter with a woven metal cylinder on the end. It looked like a tiny Chinese finger trap. He positioned it where the blockage had been and then expanded it to fit snugly against the wall of the artery. It would help prevent future clots. The whole thing only took less than an hour.

"You did great Dr. Dackel," said Hayman. "I don't know if you remember me but I was one of your students a few years ago."

"Sure I remember you," Dackel lied. "Thanks for going into cardiology and not gynecology."

On the way back to his room, he heard a voice that could only have been Deborah's coming from the ICU family area, He couldn't tell who she was speaking to, but he got the impression that she was speaking about him.

"If anything happens to him, I think I'll die," he heard her saying. They were the nicest words he ever remembered anyone ever saying about him. As he passed the lounge, he saw her standing with Red. Red looked gray. When he saw that it was Dackel, and that he was alive, the color and tone instantly returned to his face, and a single drop of salty emotion escaped from one of his tightly guarded and, thought by some to be non-existent, tear ducts.

"Buddy!" he said lunging towards the gurney shouting in a voice inappropriately loud for a football stadium, let alone a hospital, let alone an intensive care unit, "am I glad to see you, you motherfucker."

Dackel smiled. So did everyone else. They could forgive the crassness and the noise because they knew where they were coming from, and after all, this was the heart unit. Deborah raced to Dackel. She took his hand, plastic tubes, pulse oxymeter transducer and all, and squeezed it, for the first time, with love. Yes it was definitely more than concern, and positively more than relief. It was love, and they both knew it.

Chapter 34

When Sylvan Sheldon got off the plane in Tampa, he remembered why he hated Florida so much. The humidity reminded him of the days when he washed dishes in the steamy roach infested kitchen at the Family Fun Hotel in the Poconos. His glasses fogged up, he started to sweat and he found it hard to breathe. His rental car smelled mildewy and it took two minutes for the windows to de-fog. He hated the south, but not as much as he hated Jerry Edmonds and National Medical Innovations. He sped to their building.

He parked next to a rented Toyota Avalon which belonged to a very qualified video technician who just happened to walk into the personnel department looking for a position that morning. He was hired on the spot and had just finished setting up for his first assignment.

Edmonds took the precaution of having his new videographer tape the session using hidden cameras, but since he was new, he told him to set it up so that the session was recorded but not monitored in the studio.

Sheldon calmed himself down as much as he could before he went into the office.

"Mr. Edmonds," he said with a voice that still had a bit of quiver in it, "I have received some very disturbing information. I know about Alice Kirkland and I know that you had her killed. I know about Donny Moline and that you tried to kill him too. I know about the tapes that you used to threaten Dackel and how you altered the surgery tapes. I know how you ruined my marriage and how you are trying to frame me for Alice's murder. Should I go on?"

Edmonds thought for a minute. The first thing that he realized was that Donny Moline was still alive, and probably responsible for Sheldon getting the information. He considered taking the 357 out of his top desk drawer and shooting Sheldon on the spot, but he knew that would only complicate his problems. He considered denying everything, but if Sheldon came all the way down to Tampa, he must have had more than just hunches. He thought of taking the gun and killing himself. He considered that one for a while. Finally he dropped his head and said. "What do you want?"

"Fifty million," Sheldon said without blinking his beady eyes. "A check for twenty five million made out to my firm and Paul Shintock and a wire transfer of twenty five million to this bank in the Cayman Islands." He handed him a card with an account number on the back. "Fifty million and this can all go away. No more Shintock suit, no more Dackel, no suit from me for breaking up my marriage or trying to frame me. Of course you'll have to figure out how to give up Sanchez and get me off the hook, but I'm sure you'll be able to figure out a way to do that. What do you say?"

Edmonds knew he wasn't in a position to negotiate, but he also knew that even if he gave him the fifty million, it wouldn't be the end of it. He figured he would agree now and sort it out later.

"Done," he said, "give me three days."

"Twenty four hours," said Sheldon. "Fed-Ex the check to my office and call me when the transfer has been confirmed. I'll be back in Philadelphia where I can breathe." Then he got up and walked out.

Edmonds was remarkably calm considering the happenings of the last fifteen minutes. He was anything but relieved. He knew he'd never get fifty million dollars out of his insurance company and he knew he couldn't convene the board in one day. Even if he could, he couldn't tell them the whole story. And then there was Moline. He had enough information to send him to jail for a long time. And Sanchez, how could he implicate him without implicating himself? Sheldon admitted to himself that he hadn't thought this out very well.

Before he did anything else, Edmonds called his new video technician and told him to erase the tape of the meeting without viewing it. Of course before he had even gotten the call, the new technician whose name was Barry Wilson had already started to send a copy of the digitized tape over the Internet to donnym@electronet.com. A hard copy was in a Federal Express Overnight Letter Pak waiting to go. Another, labeled Best of Beavis and Butthead, was stashed inside a broken monitor.

Next, Edmonds left a message for Sanchez who was out on an assignment. He still wasn't sure what he was going to do, but he knew he had to do something and it wasn't going to have anything to do with fifty million dollars.

As soon as Donny got the tape of the meeting, he called Finney. After she saw it, she called the U.S. Attorney's office. Stacey had alerted them in advance and had already sent them a brief that documented enough to indict Edmonds and Sanchez. Now with the tape, they were sure that Sheldon would go down too.

Dackel felt great. He had no pain, the follow-up tests showed no blockage, and he felt an energy that he hadn't felt for years. He attributed it to his newly stretched coronary artery, but more likely, it came from the part of the heart that medical science has never been able to find, let alone fix. Neither he nor Deborah had said anything to each other yet, but neither had stopped talking to themselves.

When he was ready to leave the hospital, both Red and Deborah came to take him home. They both offered their homes, but he was feeling so well that he graciously turned them both down. Actually, his refusal to Red might not have sounded gracious to someone who didn't know the two of them, but it was as gracious as they ever got with each other. Dackel's exact words were, "Shit no, I'd never stay in your place, your farts are so bad your wallpaper is stained." When he heard the words, Red knew his buddy was better. He refused Deborah's offer somewhat more graciously, but he did ask that she keep Cookie for a few more weeks. She had taken her in when he first went into the hospital and Emma instantly fell in love with her. It seems that love rejuvenated Cookie too. She still couldn't see or hear very well, but she was definitely getting around better and she followed Emma everywhere.

The FBI arrested Edmonds and Sanchez in the middle of their meeting, and they took Sheldon into custody as soon as he landed in Philadelphia. The K-Mart clerk identified Sanchez as the man who bought the model rockets. That evening Sanchez hanged himself in his cell with a noose fashioned from his hair.

Because the altered tapes were never submitted into evidence in court, no charges could be filed against Edmonds for that, but he was indicted on a number of charges related to Alice Kirkland's murder and the attempted murder of Donny Moline. After thirteen months, during which time he was out on bail, and a nine-day trial, he was found not guilty on all counts. The decision outraged even the O.J. Simpson criminal trial jurors.

Since no money had actually changed hands, the charges against Sheldon were dropped, but he was disbarred for unethical behavior. His law firm pursued the lawsuit against National Medical Innovations and settled for an additional million dollars. Fourteenth Street Hospital also kicked in seven hundred thousand.

The DAC-III was sold to a well known and well respected medical equipment company who continues to train qualified physicians to use it as an alternative to hysterectomy. One of those physicians who became very skilled with the technique was Frank Andrelonis. He was one of the first to successfully use it for localized cancers of the uterus and cervix and was conducting clinical trials to study its effectiveness on stage I ovarian cancer.

Dackel's wrist got a little better and he was able to work relatively comfortably in the office but he was still unable to do surgery. His disability checks came on the fifteenth of every month.

Carlton Capuston applied to law school.

Arlene Dackel was still in a coma with no hope of recovery. Her kidneys were starting to fail and she had a stubborn pneumonia that wouldn't go away. It wouldn't be long. Dackel visited her every week.

Dackel and Deborah were seeing quite a lot of each other, and they kissed a lot, but they hadn't had sex yet. Dackel just didn't feel that it was right while his wife was still alive. Neither of them had used the "L" word yet, but they both knew it was there. She knew it instinctively. He didn't have a whole lot of instincts, so he needed more of a sign. One night, after a relaxed dinner in a quiet Italian restaurant he saw the sign, or actually, he heard it. He was walking her home and, as usual, they kissed good-bye at her door.

"I had a nice time tonight, Deborah," he said as she opened the door to her apartment.

"So did I, Al, and by the way," she said with a wink and a smile, "you can call me Debbie."

AUTHOR'S NOTE

I'M NOT DACKEL! I consider myself a pretty good surgeon and I really don't care what kind of underwear my patients wear.

My wife, Dee is not anything like Arlene, except for the fat-free lasagna which she learned to make at my request and which I'm actually pretty much getting used to. She is a beautiful, classy graceful woman of taste who does her own nails and has worked tirelessly as the president of a charitable foundation.

My children, Ellyn and Jane are sweet, affectionate, wonderful women who are mature, directed and successful. Ellyn edited my first draft and Jane was my working editor and proofreader.

My grandson Jason is the best thing on earth. Don't even try to argue.

The DAC-III is a fictional machine. I wish I had one. But for the most part, the science upon which it is based and all the other medical things I wrote about are real. Although somewhat embellished, the patient stories, even Linda Shintock's, are real too. The patient upon whom Linda's story was based was not mine, but she did die during a hysteroscopy.

And finally, a note to my patients. In these times of managed care and litigation, it is you who have kept me in medicine. Many of you have become friends even though we get to see each other only once a year. You are the best part of my job. Please, believe me when I tell you again that I'M NOT DACKEL!

Made in the USA
Monee, IL
04 November 2026

67382863R00144